Exclusive Papers of the Editorial Board Members of *Oral*

Exclusive Papers of the Editorial Board Members of *Oral*

Editors

Giuseppina Campisi
Vera Panzarella

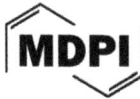

Basel • Beijing • Wuhan • Barcelona • Belgrade • Novi Sad • Cluj • Manchester

Editors
Giuseppina Campisi
University Hospital Palermo
Palermo
Italy

Vera Panzarella
University of Palermo
Palermo
Italy

Editorial Office
MDPI AG
Grosspeteranlage 5
4052 Basel, Switzerland

This is a reprint of articles from the Special Issue published online in the open access journal *Oral* (ISSN 2673-6373) (available at: https://www.mdpi.com/journal/oral/special_issues/Exclusive_Papers_EBM).

For citation purposes, cite each article independently as indicated on the article page online and as indicated below:

Lastname, A.A.; Lastname, B.B. Article Title. *Journal Name* **Year**, *Volume Number*, Page Range.

ISBN 978-3-7258-2029-0 (Hbk)
ISBN 978-3-7258-2030-6 (PDF)
doi.org/10.3390/books978-3-7258-2030-6

Cover image courtesy of Giuseppina Campisi

© 2024 by the authors. Articles in this book are Open Access and distributed under the Creative Commons Attribution (CC BY) license. The book as a whole is distributed by MDPI under the terms and conditions of the Creative Commons Attribution-NonCommercial-NoDerivs (CC BY-NC-ND) license.

Contents

Giuseppina Campisi
Editorial for Special Issue "Exclusive Papers of the Editorial Board Members of Oral"
Reprinted from: *Oral* 2024, 4, 274–281, doi:10.3390/oral4020022 1

Gianfranco Favia, Francesca Spirito, Eleonora Lo Muzio, Saverio Capodiferro, Angela Tempesta, Luisa Limongelli, et al.
Histopathological Comparative Analysis between Syndromic and Non-Syndromic Odontogenic Keratocysts: A Retrospective Study
Reprinted from: *Oral* 2022, 2, 198–204, doi:10.3390/oral2030019 9

Rita Antonelli, Oslei Paes de Almeida, Ronell Bologna-Molina and Marco Meleti
Intraoral Sialadenoma Papilliferum: A Comprehensive Review of the Literature with Emphasis on Clinical and Histopathological Diagnostic Features
Reprinted from: *Oral* 2022, 2, 242–250, doi:10.3390/oral2030023 16

Rodolfo Mauceri, Martina Coppini and Giuseppina Campisi
Onset of MRONJ in Breast Cancer Patients after Switching from Low to High Dose of Bone Modifying Agents Due to Bone Metastases Development: A Single Center Retrospective Cohort Study
Reprinted from: *Oral* 2022, 2, 274–285, doi:10.3390/oral2040026 25

Luca Testarelli, Francesca Sestito, Adriana De Stefano, Chiara Seracchiani, Roberto Vernucci and Gabriella Galluccio
Phenotypes, Genotypes, and Treatment Options of Primary Failure of Eruption: A Narrative Review
Reprinted from: *Oral* 2022, 2, 293–298, doi:10.3390/oral2040028 37

Juan José Meneu, Cecilia Fabiana Márquez-Arrico, Francisco Javier Silvestre and Javier Silvestre-Rangil
Could Periodontitis Aggravate Psoriasis?—An Update by Systematic Review
Reprinted from: *Oral* 2023, 3, 57–66, doi:10.3390/oral3010006 43

Bruno Davide Pugliese, Giovanna Garuti, Lucia Bergamini, Riccardo Karim Khamaisi, Giovanni Guaraldi, Ugo Consolo and Pierantonio Bellini
Masticatory Functionality in Post-Acute-COVID-Syndrome (PACS) Patients with and without Sarcopenia
Reprinted from: *Oral* 2023, 3, 77–91, doi:10.3390/oral3010008 53

Ourania Nicolatou-Galitis, Amanda Psyrri, Nikolaos Tsoukalas, Evangelos Galitis, Helena Linardou, Dimitra Galiti, et al.
Oral Toxicities in Cancer Patients, Who Receive Immunotherapy: A Case Series of 24 Patients
Reprinted from: *Oral* 2023, 3, 123–133, doi:10.3390/oral3010011 68

Olga Di Fede, Gaetano La Mantia, Mario G. C. A. Cimino and Giuseppina Campisi
Protection of Patient Data in Digital Oral and General Health Care: A Scoping Review with Respect to the Current Regulations
Reprinted from: *Oral* 2023, 3, 155–165, doi:10.3390/oral3020014 79

Nejat Düzgüneş, Jaroslaw Piskorz, Paulina Skupin-Mrugalska, Metin Yıldırım, Melike Sessevmez and Jennifer Cheung
Photodynamic Therapy of Oral Cancer and Novel Liposomal Photosensitizers
Reprinted from: *Oral* 2023, 3, 276–294, doi:10.3390/oral3030023 90

Antonio Manni, Stefano Pera, Giorgio Gastaldi, Andrea Boggio and Mauro Cozzani
Skeletal Anchorage in Treating Skeletal Class II Malocclusion in Growing Patients Using the Herbst Appliance
Reprinted from: *Oral* **2023**, *3*, 539–544, doi:10.3390/oral3040044 . . . . **109**

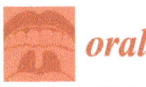 *oral*

Editorial

Editorial for Special Issue "Exclusive Papers of the Editorial Board Members of Oral"

Giuseppina Campisi

Department of Rehabilitation, Fragility and Continuity of Care, Unit of Oral Medicine, University Hospital Palermo, 90127 Palermo, Italy; campisi@policlinico.pa.it

Citation: Campisi, G. Editorial for Special Issue "Exclusive Papers of the Editorial Board Members of Oral". *Oral* **2024**, *4*, 274–281. https://doi.org/10.3390/oral4020022

Received: 11 June 2024
Accepted: 13 June 2024
Published: 18 June 2024

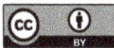

Copyright: © 2024 by the author. Licensee MDPI, Basel, Switzerland. This article is an open access article distributed under the terms and conditions of the Creative Commons Attribution (CC BY) license (https://creativecommons.org/licenses/by/4.0/).

1. Introduction

In 2022, the World Health Organization (WHO) released a landmark report on oral health, emphasizing the staggering global prevalence of oral disorders, which affect approximately 3.5 billion individuals [1]. These conditions are among the most widespread noncommunicable diseases, significantly burdening low- and middle-income nations. The report underscores that oral health is vital not only for fundamental functions such as breathing, speaking, and eating but also for people's overall health, well-being, and social confidence.

Despite its critical importance, oral health is constantly threatened by a range of diseases and conditions, compounded by significant disparities in the cost and accessibility of care. Marginalized and disadvantaged populations are particularly vulnerable to these issues. The WHO report highlights that many oral illnesses can be effectively treated and prevented with affordable measures. Strategies that address common risk factors among noncommunicable diseases are especially promising, particularly in resource-constrained settings.

To address these challenges, it is essential to have a well-trained and adequately staffed dental workforce and to integrate oral health services into universal health coverage plans, ensuring that these services are both accessible and affordable.

Specialized journals such as *Oral* from MDPI play a crucial role in advancing this mission by promoting and disseminating research across a broad spectrum of oral health topics. This Special Issue exemplifies the Editorial Board's dedication to exploring a diverse range of critical areas, each contributing valuable insights into the field.

The studies in this Issue cover a wide array of topics, reflecting the heterogeneity and complexity of oral health. They include comparative histopathological analyses that deepen our understanding of disease mechanisms, reviews of rare benign tumors that inform diagnostic and therapeutic strategies, and investigations into medication-related osteonecrosis that highlight the intersection between oral health and systemic disease. Additionally, the Issue addresses primary failure of eruption, the interplay between periodontal disease and systemic conditions, the impact of post-acute COVID-19 syndrome on oral function, and oral complications arising from cancer therapies. Furthermore, it explores the transformative potential of digital health technologies in oral care, the innovative use of photodynamic therapy in treating oral cancers, and novel approaches to orthodontic challenges.

The breadth of these topics underscores the necessity of comprehensive research to address the multifaceted nature of oral health. By delving into these diverse areas, the studies contribute to a deeper understanding of oral health, inform clinical practice, and ultimately aim to improve patient outcomes. The commitment to such a wide-ranging exploration of oral health issues is both timely and essential for advancing the field and addressing the significant global burden of oral diseases.

With this vision in mind, some of the Editorial Board members of *Oral* have made scientific contributions to this Special Issue. Here, we present an overview of these published articles, showcasing this diverse and impactful research aimed at advancing the field of oral health. Their dedication to and passion for addressing these critical topics are evident, and their contributions significantly enhance our understanding and approach to improving oral health worldwide.

2. Overview of Studies

The study by Favia et al. (contribution 1) explores the efficacy of carrying out a comparative histopathological analysis between syndromic and non-syndromic odontogenic keratocysts (OKs), employing both conventional and Confocal Laser Scanning Microscopy (CLSM). Their investigation reveals some of the distinctive features of syndromic OKs, including increased satellite cysts, a basophilic layer in the basement membrane, and heightened cellular activity, as detected by CLSM. These findings suggest a potential correlation between histopathological characteristics and the biological behavior of OKs, particularly in terms of recurrence rates. The authors conclude that CLSM represents a valuable technology for distinguishing between syndromic and non-syndromic OKs, aiding the precise prediction of their biological behavior. This could facilitate tailored clinical and radiological follow-ups for patients. Notably, the study underscores the importance of novel histopathological findings, particularly those identified through CLSM, in advancing our understanding and the early diagnosis of conditions like Nevoid Basal Cell Carcinoma Syndrome (NBCCS), where OKs may serve as an initial manifestation.

The study's strengths lie in its comprehensive approach, combining conventional histopathology with advanced imaging techniques, and its focus on clinically relevant outcomes, such as recurrence rates. However, the authors acknowledge various limitations, such as the absence of discrimination between orthokeratinized and parakeratinized keratocysts and the lack of correlation with immunohistochemical analyses. Despite these limitations, the study advocates for the potential integration of CLSM as a supplementary tool in oral pathology, offering insights into the molecular and morphological distinctions between syndromic and sporadic OKs.

Antonelli et al. (contribution 2) conducted a comprehensive review of intraoral sialadenoma papilliferum (SP), a rare benign epithelial tumor originating from the salivary gland. Published in *Oral* in 2022, the study aims to elucidate the clinical and histopathological diagnostic features of this condition. SP was first described in 1969 and poses diagnostic challenges due to its rarity. The review analyzed 64 reported cases, highlighting the fact that SP predominantly affects males with a mean age of 57.2 years. The most common site is the palate, often presenting as a slow-growing, asymptomatic papillary lesion. Histologically, SP exhibits characteristic features such as papillary projections lined by two or three layers of cells. Treatment typically involves conservative excision. Despite concerns about malignant transformation, SP is generally considered to be a benign neoplasm with low recurrence rates. However, a few cases with uncertain malignant features have been reported, warranting further research to clarify their biological behavior and histogenesis. The authors conclude that SP, though rare, should be considered in the differential diagnosis of intraoral swellings, particularly those located on the palate, and advocate for more studies to understand its biology better.

The retrospective cohort study conducted by Mauceri et al. (contribution 3) investigates the onset of Medication-Related Osteonecrosis of the Jaw (MRONJ) in breast cancer (BC) patients following a switch from low doses (LD) to high doses (HD) of bone-modifying agents (BMAs) due to the development of bone metastases. The study outlines the prevalence of MRONJ, primarily associated with BMAs, in the context of breast cancer therapy, which often leads to cancer treatment-induced bone loss (CTIBL) necessitating LD-BMAs treatment. The objectives include describing the characteristics of BC patients undergoing treatment with LD-BMAs for CTIBL prevention, documenting any transitions to HD-BMAs, assessing the occurrence of MRONJ, and identifying potential associated risk factors. Fourteen female BC patients with a mean age of 66.6 years receiving LD-BMAs for CTIBL prevention were included in the study. Among them, four patients were switched to HD-BMAs due to bone metastases. Intriguingly, MRONJ developed in two of these patients: one in the mandible after being on risedronate followed by denosumab (HD) and the other in the maxilla after denosumab (LD) followed by zoledronate treatment. The authors conclude that BC patients undergoing treatment with LD-BMAs for CTIBL may face a MRONJ risk similar to osteo-metabolic patients. Therefore, meticulous monitoring of oral health is recommended for these individuals, especially considering the potential transition from LD to HD BMA therapies for bone metastasis, which can increase the risk of MRONJ.

This research sheds light on the importance of vigilant oral health surveillance and risk assessment in BC patients undergoing BMA therapy, particularly in the context of treatment adjustments for bone metastases, to mitigate the potential occurrence of MRONJ.

In their narrative review, Testarelli et al. (contribution 4) explore the clinical, genetic, and therapeutic aspects of primary failure of eruption (PFE), a condition characterized by incomplete tooth eruption despite a clear pathway. The authors conducted a comprehensive literature search, summarizing findings from 12 relevant articles published between 2008 and June 2022. The authors highlight the predominance of genotypical discussions (ten out of twelve articles) concerning PFE, emphasizing the role of PTH1R mutations in disrupting the balance between bone resorption and apposition during tooth eruption. Phenotypical aspects and epidemiological data were also discussed, but treatment options received less attention, with only three out of the twelve articles addressing this aspect.

The review investigates epidemiological variations in PFE prevalence and gender distribution, emphasizing the need for further research to clarify these disparities. It identifies distinct PFE types based on eruption potential and distribution patterns. Additionally, the review underscores the familial inheritance of PFE, particularly mutations in the PTH1R gene, affecting calcium metabolism and bone resorption. Testarelli et al. advocate for a differential diagnosis between PFE and other conditions to inform appropriate treatment strategies. They emphasize the importance of PTH1R screening before orthodontic interventions to mitigate the risk of ankylosis and iatrogenic damage. However, the review acknowledges that there is a dearth of information on treatment modalities, stressing the necessity for future studies to guide effective therapeutic approaches tailored to individual patients.

The fifth text published in this Special Issue is a systematic review by Meneu et al. (contribution 5) on the potential aggravating effect of periodontitis on psoriasis. Psoriasis, a chronic inflammatory disease, has been associated with periodontal pathologies, particularly periodontitis. The aim of the study was to determine if periodontitis could exacerbate psoriasis. Following the PRISMA guidelines, the authors conducted a comprehensive systematic review, employing a PECO (Participants, Exposure, Control, and Outcomes) question model. They searched various databases and identified 111 studies, of which 11 met the inclusion criteria. These comprised nine case-control studies, one cross-sectional study, and one cohort study. Most studies reported an increase in bleeding on probing and the presence of periodontal pockets in patients with psoriasis, suggesting that local periodontal inflammation could aggravate psoriasis. The included studies evaluated various periodontal parameters such as probing depth (PD), clinical attachment loss (CAL), and the community periodontal index of treatment need (CPITN). While some studies found differences in these parameters between psoriasis patients and controls, the results were not consistent across all studies. The prevalence and the incidence rates of periodontitis were higher among psoriasis patients compared to controls in several studies, indicating a potential association between psoriasis and periodontal disease. The systematic review concludes that periodontitis could aggravate the clinical manifestations of psoriasis. The bidirectional association between the two conditions is attributed to shared immunological, microbiological, and environmental factors. The findings highlight the importance of dental examination and treatment in patients with psoriasis to improve systemic inflammatory processes and potentially mitigate the progression of psoriasis.

Pugliese et al. (contribution 6) aimed to investigate masticatory function levels in post-acute-COVID-syndrome (PACS) patients with and without sarcopenia. The study included twenty-three PACS patients, among whom thirteen suffered from sarcopenia, five complained of asthenia without sarcopenia, and five had neither muscle symptoms nor asthenia. Masticatory strength and effectiveness were assessed using a gnathodynamometer and a chewing gum mixing ability test, respectively. Additionally, hand grip and gait speed tests were conducted. The findings revealed that PACS sarcopenic patients exhibited decreased masticatory effectiveness and strength compared to asthenic non-sarcopenic patients and non-asthenic non-sarcopenic patients. The study also explored medical history, anatomo-functional analysis, intra-oral examination, and bite force measurement. Notably, the research suggested a correlation between oral health, particularly the number of teeth and the DMFT index, and masticatory performance in PACS patients. Despite the limitations, including the lack of pre-COVID-19 chewing performance data and the small sample size, the study underscores the importance of addressing oral health issues in PACS patients through a multidisciplinary rehabilitation approach. Further research with larger cohorts is recommended to validate these findings and assess the clinical utility of the gnathodynamometer as a bite force measurement tool.

Authored by Nicolatou-Galitis et al. (contribution 7), the seventh study in this Special Issue investigates the oral complications experienced by 24 patients with cancer who underwent immunotherapy between 2017 and 2022. The average age of the patients was 64 years, with lung cancer being the most prevalent form of cancer within the cohort. During immunotherapy, the patients presented with various symptoms, including oral pain, xerostomia, burning sensations, and gingival bleeding. Notably, immune-related lesions affected 62.5% of the patients, with three cases exacerbating pre-existing autoimmune diseases. Moreover, six cases of oral infections and six cases of medication-related osteonecrosis of the jaw were identified, highlighting the multifaceted nature of oral complications in immunotherapy. Of significance is the observation that patients previously or concurrently treated with other anticancer therapies appeared to be at a higher risk of experiencing oral issues. The findings of Nicolatou-Galitis et al. underscore the importance of vigilant monitoring and management of oral health during immunotherapy, emphasizing the need for multidisciplinary collaboration among oncologists, dentists, and other healthcare professionals. Understanding the potential oral complications associated with immunotherapy is essential for optimizing patient care and outcomes in the rapidly evolving landscape of cancer treatment.

The article authored by Di Fede et al. (contribution 8) inquiries into the increasingly critical role of digital health technologies, such as telemedicine and teledentistry, in modern healthcare, particularly accentuated by the SARS-CoV-2 pandemic. These technologies offer significant advantages in terms of reducing healthcare provider workload and enhancing patient outcomes, especially in scenarios requiring remote monitoring, diagnosis, and communication. However, alongside these benefits, concerns regarding clinical risks, data security, and privacy protection have emerged. The paper conducts a scoping review, following the PRISMA-ScR guidelines and Arksey and O'Malley's five-step framework, to explore the regulatory landscape surrounding the utilization of digital health apps and software in healthcare. Examining 24 selected articles, the review highlights a predominant focus on data security policies within the healthcare industry, underscoring the necessity for robust regulations and app control systems to safeguard patient data effectively. Moreover, the review identifies a pressing need for enhanced research efforts and policy initiatives to bolster data security practices and address privacy and safety challenges associated with health-related apps. Notably, inconsistencies in standards regarding professional obligation and informed consent in online medical consultations are noted, posing risks concerning data privacy, medical liabilities, and ethical considerations. Despite the transformative potential of digital health in revolutionizing medical service delivery, the article underscores existing challenges, including the absence of standardized protocols for handling sensitive patient data and the lack of uniform legislative provisions. These deficiencies raise significant concerns regarding confidentiality and security in digital healthcare ecosystems. The authors emphasize the critical importance of regulatory compliance to elucidate and harmonize regulations, providing clear guidelines for healthcare practitioners and the broader health system. Ultimately, the article advocates for urgent regulatory measures aimed at regulating patient data, clarifying provisions, and promoting informed patient participation to maximize the efficacy and successful implementation of telemedicine practices.

In their comprehensive study, Düzgüneş et al. (contribution 9) examine the effectiveness of photodynamic therapy (PDT) in treating oral cancer, with a particular emphasis on novel liposomal photosensitizers. They highlight the advantages of PDT, which utilizes a combination of a photosensitizer drug, specific light wavelengths, and oxygen to selectively destroy cancerous tissues. The study reviews several photosensitizers, including Methylene Blue, 5-aminolevulinic acid (the precursor to protoporphyrin IX), porphyrin, Foscan, Chlorin e6, and HPPH, all of which have demonstrated success in treating oral verrucous hyperplasia, oral leukoplakia, oral lichen planus, and head and neck squamous cell carcinoma. The authors emphasize the potential of "theranostic" liposomes, which combine diagnostic and therapeutic functions by delivering both a contrast agent for magnetic resonance imaging (MRI) and a photosensitizer for image-guided PDT of head and neck cancer. These liposomes can be targeted to cancer cells by incorporating photosensitizers that specifically bind to cell surface markers overexpressed on these cells. A significant advancement discussed in the study is the development of novel porphyrinoids in the authors' laboratories. When encapsulated in cationic liposomes, these compounds exhibit up to 50 times lower IC50 values compared to their free counterparts, indicating a markedly increased potency. The study concludes that the targeted delivery of photosensitizers using liposomal encapsulation significantly enhances the effectiveness of PDT for oral cancers. The innovative approach of using theranostic liposomes and novel porphy-rinoids shows promise for improving the precision and efficacy of cancer treatment. The authors foresee those further advancements, such as targeting cancer stem cells and utilizing upconversion nanoparticles for near-infrared irradiation, will overcome current limitations like tumor hypoxia, thereby enhancing the overall therapeutic outcomes of PDT for tumors accessible to light sources. This research highlights the potential of integrating advanced drug delivery systems with photodynamic therapy to achieve more effective and targeted treatment modalities for oral and head and neck cancers.

The opinion article by Matti et al. (contribution 10) provides insights into the efficacy of treating skeletal Class II malocclusion. They highlight the efficiency of the Herbst appliance while emphasizing the need to control undesired dental movements that may affect orthopedic outcomes. The introduction of skeletal anchorage, through the use of miniscrews and elastic ligatures, allows for better control over unwanted dental movements, thus enhancing the treatment's effectiveness. Moreover, skeletal anchorage offers the opportunity to selectively correct various components of Class II malocclusion, paving the way for a new diagnostic approach that prioritizes facial aesthetics over occlusal relations. This approach relies on the aesthetic evaluation of the patient, with particular attention to the nasolabial angle, lips, and sagittal position of the maxilla and mandible. The treatment of skeletal Class II malocclusion requires a specific focus on patient aesthetics. The combination of the Herbst appliance, elastic ligatures, and skeletal anchorage represents an effective therapeutic option. However, further well-designed randomized clinical trials are needed to confirm the long-term results of this treatment approach.

3. Conclusions

In conclusion, this Special Issue of *Oral* highlights the remarkable breadth and depth of contemporary research into oral health. The contributions from our esteemed Editorial Board Members underscore the critical importance of addressing diverse and complex challenges within the field.

A Special Issue in a scientific journal often benefits from a unifying theme or guiding principle. While selecting a specific theme may attract experts in that field, opting for a guiding principle can intrigue a broader readership. In this regard, our approach has been to emphasize topics related to oral soft and hard tissue diseases, anchored in a forward-looking perspective that integrates advanced diagnostics and the promotion of preventive and therapeutic principles. We aimed to address issues relevant to diverse segments of the population while also providing exemplars for the broader scientific community. This over-arching principle underscores our commitment to advancing oral health research and practice in the contemporary era.

The articles featured in this Special Issue offer profound implications for both clinical practice and research in the field of oral health. The comparative histopathological analysis conducted by Favia et al. not only distinguishes features between syndromic and non-syndromic OKs but also provides valuable insights into their biological behavior and recurrence rates. This suggests the potential of CLSM as a diagnostic tool, enabling more precise predictions and tailored follow-up strategies for patients, thereby enhancing clinical management. Similarly, Antonelli et al.'s comprehensive review of intraoral SP elucidates the clinical and histopathological features of this rare benign tumor, guiding clinicians in appropriate diagnostic and management approaches.

Mauceri et al.'s retrospective cohort study highlights the importance of vigilant monitoring of breast cancer patients undergoing BMA therapy to mitigate the risk of MRONJ. This underscores the necessity for meticulous oral health surveillance and risk assessment, especially in the context of treatment adjustments for bone metastases, thus informing clinical decision making and patient management strategies.

The narrative review by Testarelli et al. emphasizes the significance of differential diagnosis and PTH1R screening in guiding treatment strategies for PFE, thereby enhancing clinical management approaches. Furthermore, the systematic review by Meneu et al. underscores the bidirectional association between periodontitis and psoriasis, highlighting the importance of dental examination and treatment in patients with psoriasis to mitigate systemic inflammatory processes and improve patient outcomes.

Additionally, Pugliese et al.'s study emphasizes the correlation between oral health and masticatory performance in PACS patients, advocating for multidisciplinary rehabilitation approaches to address oral health issues in this population, thus informing rehabilitative strategies for PACS patients.

Nicolatou-Galitis et al.'s investigation into oral complications in cancer patients undergoing immunotherapy emphasizes the need for vigilant monitoring and multidisciplinary collaboration to optimize patient care and outcomes. Furthermore, the study by Di Fede et al. highlights the increasingly critical role of digital health technologies, such as telemedicine and teledentistry, in modern healthcare, which has been accentuated by the SARS-CoV-2 pandemic in particular. These technologies offer significant advantages in terms of reducing healthcare provider workload and enhancing patient outcomes, especially in scenarios requiring remote monitoring, diagnosis, and communication. However, alongside these benefits, concerns regarding clinical risks, data security, and privacy protection have emerged.

Finally, Düzgüneş et al.'s study on the use of PDT in treating oral cancer underscores the potential of novel liposomal photosensitizers in enhancing the effectiveness of PDT for oral cancers. These findings collectively underscore the necessity of comprehensive research to inform clinical practice, optimize patient care, and ultimately improve oral health outcomes worldwide.

All of these studies collectively emphasize the urgent need for continued investment in oral health research, particularly in the context of global health disparities. As evidenced by the topics covered, oral health is inextricably linked to overall well-being, and advancements in this area can have profound implications for public health. By focusing on a wide array of issues—from the impact of systemic diseases on oral health to innovative treatments and the integration of digital health technologies—the research in this Issue provides a comprehensive overview of the current state and future directions of oral health.

The dedication and passion of our contributors are palpable, reflecting a shared commitment to improving patient outcomes and advancing the field. Their work not only enhances our scientific understanding but also paves the way for improved clinical practices and policies that can better address the global burden of oral diseases.

As we move forward, it is essential to foster collaboration among researchers, clinicians, and policymakers to translate these scientific insights into tangible health benefits. The findings and discussions presented in this Issue of *Oral* are a testament to the power of scientific inquiry and its potential to drive meaningful change in the field of oral health.

We hope that this Special Issue will inspire further research, encourage multidisciplinary collaboration, and ultimately contribute to a future where oral health is universally recognized and prioritized as a fundamental component of overall health and well-being.

Acknowledgments: Many thanks to Fortunato Buttacavoli, at University of Palermo, for his valuable assistance and support.

Conflicts of Interest: The author declare no conflict of interest.

List of Contributions:

1. Favia, G.; Spirito, F.; Lo Muzio, E.; Capodiferro, S.; Tempesta, A.; Limongelli, L.; Lo Muzio, L.; Maiorano, E. Histopathological Comparative Analysis between Syndromic and Non-Syndromic Odontogenic Keratocysts: A Retrospective Study. *Oral* **2022**, *2*, 198–204. https://doi.org/10.3390/oral2030019.
2. Antonelli, R.; Paes de Almeida, O.; Bologna-Molina, R.; Meleti, M. Intraoral Sialadenoma Papilliferum: A Comprehensive Review of the Literature with Emphasis on Clinical and Histopathological Diagnostic Features. *Oral* **2022**, *2*, 242–250. https://doi.org/10.3390/oral2030023.
3. Mauceri, R.; Coppini, M.; Campisi, G. Onset of MRONJ in Breast Cancer Patients after Switching from Low to High Dose of Bone Modifying Agents Due to Bone Metastases Development: A Single Center Retrospective Cohort Study. *Oral* **2022**, *2*, 274–285. https://doi.org/10.3390/oral2040026.
4. Testarelli, L.; Sestito, F.; De Stefano, A.; Seracchiani, C.; Vernucci, R.; Galluccio, G. Phenotypes, Genotypes, and Treatment Options of Primary Failure of Eruption: A Narrative Review. *Oral* **2022**, *2*, 293–298. https://doi.org/10.3390/oral2040028.
5. Meneu, J.; Márquez-Arrico, C.; Silvestre, F.; Silvestre-Rangil, J. Could Periodontitis Aggravate Psoriasis?—An Update by Systematic Review. *Oral* **2023**, *3*, 57–66. https://doi.org/10.3390/oral3010006.
6. Pugliese, B.; Garuti, G.; Bergamini, L.; Khamaisi, R.; Guaraldi, G.; Consolo, U.; Bellini, P. Masticatory Func-tionality in Post-Acute-COVID-Syndrome (PACS) Patients with and without Sarcopenia. *Oral* **2023**, *3*, 77–91. https://doi.org/10.3390/oral3010008.
7. Nicolatou-Galitis, O.; Psyrri, A.; Tsoukalas, N.; Galitis, E.; Linardou, H.; Galiti, D.; Athansiadis, I.; Kalapanida, D.; Razis, E.; Katirtzoglou, N.; Kentepozidis, N.; Kosmidis, P.; Stavridi, F.; Kyrodimos, E.; Daliani, D.; Tsironis, G.; Mountzios, G.; Karageorgopoulou, S.; Gouveris, P.; Syrigos, K. Oral Toxicities in Cancer Patients, Who Receive Immunotherapy: A Case Series of 24 Patients. *Oral* **2023**, *3*, 123–133. https://doi.org/10.3390/oral3010011.
8. Di Fede, O.; La Mantia, G.; Cimino, M.; Campisi, G. Protection of Patient Data in Digital Oral and General Health Care: A Scoping Review with Respect to the Current Regulations. *Oral* **2023**, *3*, 155–165. https://doi.org/10.3390/oral3020014.
9. Düzgüneş, N.; Piskorz, J.; Skupin-Mrugalska, P.; Yıldırım, M.; Sessevmez, M.; Cheung, J. Photodynamic Therapy of Oral Cancer and Novel Liposomal Photosensitizers. *Oral* **2023**, *3*, 276–294. https://doi.org/10.3390/oral3030023.
10. Manni, A.; Pera, S.; Gastaldi, G.; Boggio, A.; Cozzani, M. Skeletal Anchorage in Treating Skeletal Class II Malocclusion in Growing Patients Using the Herbst Appliance. *Oral* **2023**, *3*, 539–544. https://doi.org/10.3390/oral3040044.

Reference

1. Global Oral Health Status Report: Towards Universal Health Coverage for Oral Health by 2030. Available online: https://www.who.int/publications/i/item/9789240061484 (accessed on 5 June 2024).

Disclaimer/Publisher's Note: The statements, opinions and data contained in all publications are solely those of the individual author(s) and contributor(s) and not of MDPI and/or the editor(s). MDPI and/or the editor(s) disclaim responsibility for any injury to people or property resulting from any ideas, methods, instructions or products referred to in the content.

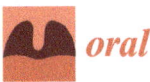

Article

Histopathological Comparative Analysis between Syndromic and Non-Syndromic Odontogenic Keratocysts: A Retrospective Study

Gianfranco Favia [1], Francesca Spirito [2], Eleonora Lo Muzio [3], Saverio Capodiferro [1], Angela Tempesta [1], Luisa Limongelli [1], Lorenzo Lo Muzio [2,4,*] and Eugenio Maiorano [5]

1 Odontostomatology Unit, Department of Interdisciplinary Medicine, Faculty of Dental Medicine, "Aldo Moro" University of Bari, p.za G. Cesare 11, 70124 Bari, Italy; gianfranco.favia@uniba.it (G.F.); capodiferro.saverio@gmail.com (S.C.); angela.tempesta1989@gmail.com (A.T.); luisanna.limongelli@gmail.com (L.L.)
2 Department of Clinical and Experimental Medicine, Dental School, University of Foggia, Via Rovelli 50, 71122 Foggia, Italy; francesca.spirito@unifg.it
3 Department of Translational Medicine and for Romagna, School of Orthodontics, University of Ferrara, Via Luigi Borsari 46, 44121 Ferrara, Italy; eleonoralomuzio@gmail.com
4 Consorzio Interuniversitario Nazionale per la Bio-Oncologia (CINBO),Via dei Vestini 31, 66100 Chieti, Italy
5 Pathological Anatomy Unit, Department of Emergency and Organ Transplantation, Faculty of Medicine, "Aldo Moro" University of Bari, p.za G. Cesare 11, 70124 Bari, Italy; eugenio.maiorano@uniba.it
* Correspondence: lorenzo.lomuzio@unifg.it; Tel.: +390881588090

Abstract: (1) Background: The aim of this study was to compare the histopathological features of syndromic and non-syndromic odontogenic keratocysts (OKs) using conventional and Confocal Laser Scanning Microscopy (CLSM) with their biological behaviour. (2) Methods: Data from the medical records of 113 patients with histological diagnosis of (single and/or multiple) OKs were collected. Globally, 213 OKs (120 syndromic and 93 sporadic) were retrieved, and their histological slides were re-evaluated with conventional H&E staining and with autofluorescence on the same slides using CLSM (Nikon Eclipse E600 microscope). (3) Results: Syndromic OKs showed more satellite cysts than sporadic cases, as well as a basophilic layer in the basement membrane, which was absent in sporadic OKs; both were highlighted with CLSM. The basement membrane in syndromic OKs appeared amorphous and fragile, thus possibly being responsible for the epithelial detachment and collapse, with scalloped features. Furthermore, the basal epithelial layers in such cases also showed increased cellularity and proliferative activity. All these histological features may possibly justify their higher tendency to recur. (4) Conclusions: CLSM is useful advanced technology that could help to quickly and easily discriminate between syndromic and non-syndromic OKs and to more accurately predict their biological behaviour in order to set fitter clinico-radiological follow-ups for individual patients.

Keywords: odontogenic keratocyst; Nevoid Basal-Cell Carcinoma Syndrome; Gorlin Syndrome; Confocal Laser Scanning Microscope; jaws; oral diseases

1. Introduction

The odontogenic keratocyst (OK) was first described in 1956 by Philpsen as an odontogenic cyst with keratinized epithelium [1], and later, because of its aggressive behaviour, high recurrence rates, and specific histological characteristics [2], it was re-classified as "a benign uni- or multi-cystic, intra-osseus tumour of odontogenic origin (Keratocystic odontogenic tumour-KCOT), with a characteristic lining of para-keratinized stratified squamous epithelium and potential for aggressive, infiltrative behaviour" by the World Health Organization (WHO) in 2005 [3]. In the 2017 classification of head and neck tumours, this pathological entity was reverted back from tumour to the original and well-accepted terminology of odontogenetic keratocyst [4], because despite the characteristics of aggressive growth, post-operative recurrence, the rare reports of solid variants of OKs, and mutations in the PTCH gene, there was not sufficient evidence to support the classification as a tumour [5].

In the newest 2022 edition of the WHO classification of head and neck tumours, the OK continues to be part of the cyst classification [6].

It may be solitary or multiple and occur synchronously or metachronously in one or both jaws, the latter being considered as one stigmata of the inherited Nevoid Basal-Cell Carcinoma Syndrome (NBCCS) [3]. NBCCS is a rare genetic condition with an autosomal-dominant inheritance pattern, showing variable expressiveness and complete penetrance, firstly defined in 1960 by Gorlin and Goltz as a condition including multiple basal-cell nevi, multiple OKs, and skeletal abnormalities [7].

OKs can occur in wide age range, with a peak in the third and fourth decades and a second smaller peak in the elderly with a slight male predilection [8] (the reported male–female ratio is 1.6:1 [2]). OKs are believed to arise from the dental lamina or its remnants, which include the pre-functional lamina, not involved in tooth formation [9], and occasionally, from the basal layers of the overlying mucosa [10].

Several studies have highlighted the role of the PTCH1 gene in the aetiology of both syndromic and sporadic OKs. The PTCH1 gene, mapped on chromosome 9q22.3-q31, encodes for a transmembrane receptor for Sonic Hedgehog (SHH). The PTCH–SHH pathway is involved in the pathogenesis of sporadic and syndromic tumours (associated with NBCCS), such as OKs, basal-cell carcinomas, medulloblastomas, and trichoepitheliomas [11].

OKs more frequently involve the angle of the mandible (the mandible–maxilla ratio is 2:1) [12]. These tumours may reach a large size prior to identification, and patients may complain of pain, swelling, or discharge in almost 60% of the cases [13]. Radiographically, an OK may appear as a small and round unilocular radiolucency or may be larger and multilocular with scalloped margins. In 25–40% of cases, OKs may be present in association with impacted or displaced teeth, whereas dental root erosion rarely occurs [14].

Typically, histologic findings of OKs show a para-keratinized stratified squamous epithelium, usually 5–8-cell-layer thick, which demarcates a cystic lumen filled with desquamated keratin [2]. There is a well-defined, often palisaded, basal layer of columnar or cuboidal cells, whereas the parakeratotic cells in the upper layers often show a corrugated surface. Satellite cysts may be seen in the surrounding fibrous connective tissues. Occasionally, epithelial dysplasia may be present, but the malignant transformation to squamous-cell carcinoma is exceedingly rare [4].

Another, less frequent histologic variant was described, i.e., the orthokeratinized odontogenic keratocyst [15]. In this case, histology is characterized by thin, uniform, orthokeratinized lining epithelium with an onion-skin-like luminal surface keratinization, prominent stratum granulosum, and low cuboidal or flattened basal-cell layer with little tendency of nuclear palisading [16].

When OKs show features such as small satellite cysts or solid islands in the cystic wall or budding of the basal layer, they are generally associated with NBCCS [4].

Patients with syndromic keratocysts may be at greater risk for developing more numerous and severe BCCs and other neoplastic growths, including ovarian fibromas [17].

The aim of this study was to report on novel histopathological findings, as detected with Confocal Laser Scanning Microscopy (CLSM), and to compare such findings with the biological behaviour of both syndromic and sporadic OKs in order to determine specific features that could facilitate the early diagnosis of NBCCS in those patients where the first manifestation is that of OKs.

2. Materials and Methods

This retrospective study was performed at Odontostomatology and Surgery Unit of University of Bari Aldo Moro.

The current study was carried out in accordance with the principles of the Declaration of Helsinki; in addition, it was approved by the institutional review board (study No. 4599, Prot. 1528/C.E.); patients released informed consent for diagnostic/therapeutic procedures and for the possible use of the biologic samples for research purposes.

In the period between 1979 and 2020, a total number of 126 patients were histologically diagnosed with 228 syndromic and sporadic OKs. All patients provided written informed consent before any study-related procedure was started.

All samples were fixed in 10% neutral-buffered formalin, paraffin-embedded, thin-sectioned at 3–4 μm, and stained with haematoxylin–eosin. All histological slides were re-evaluated using a Nikon Eclipse E600 microscope (Nikon Corporation, Tokio, Japan), equipped with argon and helium–neon lasers emitting at 488–543-nm wavelengths, which allowed us to perform both optical and Confocal Laser Scanning Microscope (CLSM) analyses. Nikon EZ C1 software (ver. 2.10; Nikon Corporation, Coord Automatizing) was used for bidimensional image processing. For each sample, ten 512 × 512 × 12-bit bidimensional images were acquired.

Following histological re-evaluation, 13 patients harbouring 15 OKs were excluded due to equivocal morphologic presentation, which did not allow us to definitely rule out cysts of other types. Overall, 213 OKs from 113 patients were included in this study. The collected data included gender, age at diagnosis, familiarity in syndromic patients, site, size, multiplicity, maxillary-sinus involvement, associated impacted teeth, treatment modalities, and recurrence rate. The chi-squared test (χ^2) was used to detect associations between the several analysed variables using a 95% significance level ($p < 0.05$).

3. Results

The main clinic–radiological features of the investigated patients are summarized in Table 1. Overall, 31 patients were affected by NBCCS (group 1), while the remaining 82 patients presented sporadic (non-syndromic) lesions (group 2). In group 1, the age range was 3.5–53 years, whereas in group 2, it was 9–86 years. Interestingly, OKs were detected in a larger cohort of paediatric patients (18 years old or younger) ($n = 11/31 = 35.48\%$) of group 1 in comparison with those of group 2 ($n = 9/82 = 10.98\%$), this difference being statistically significant ($\chi^2 = 9.28$; $p = 0.0023$).

Table 1. Clinical data of the 113 patients included in this study.

	Syndromic Patients		Sporadic Patients	
	N	%	N	%
	31	27.43%	82	72.57%
Males	19	61.29%	49	59.76%
Females	12	38.71%	33	40.24%
Male–female ratio	1.48:1		1.58:1	
Age range	3.5–53		9–86	
Mean age	25.79 ± 14.46 SD		38.99 ± 18.98 SD	
Paediatric patients	11	35.48%	9	10.98%
Lesions	120		93	
Mandibular lesions	79	65.83%	80	86.02%
Maxillary lesions	41	34.17%	13	13.98%
Mandible–maxilla ratio	1.9:1		5.8:1	
Major lesions (diameter > 3 cm)	68	56.67%	50	53.76%
Multiple lesions	23	19.17%	0	0%
Associated impacted teeth	31	25.83%	12	12.9%
Patients with recurrences	12	38.71%	8	9.76%

N: number of patients. %: percentage of patients

The male–female ratio was almost 1.5:1 in both groups. Both sporadic and syndromic OKs preferentially involved the mandible rather than the maxilla (the mandible–maxilla ratio was 1.9:1 in syndromic OKs and 5.8:1 in sporadic lesions), and 20.19% of the lesions were associated with impacted teeth.

Within group 1, 74.19% of the patients presented multiple lesions (81 OKs = 3.52/patient), while no multiple lesions were identified among patients of group 2 ($\chi^2 = 76.39$; $p < 0.0001$).

In addition, following conservative surgery, 12 syndromic patients experienced 26 recurrences (38.71%; $n = 12/31$), as opposed to 8 patients with sporadic OKs who presented 11 recurrences (9.76%; $n = 8/82$) ($\chi^2 = 12.95$; $p = 0.0003$).

The histological findings are summarized in Table 2. Syndromic OKs analysed with CLSM presented more numerous satellite cysts, due to the budding of the basal-cell layers in the underlying connective tissue, than sporadic lesions (Figure 1A,B). Furthermore, the epithelial layers appeared more densely cellular and more intensely mitotically active in syndromic OKs, in comparison with sporadic cases. Interestingly, a subepithelial basophilic layer was clearly detectable in syndromic OKs (Figure 1C,D) and absent in non-syndromic OKs (Figure 1E,F). Moreover, the basement membrane in syndromic OKs resulted amorphous and fragile, this feature being possibly responsible for the detachment of the epithelial component, which appeared collapsed and ramified, with a scalloped and corrugated aspect (Figure 1G,H).

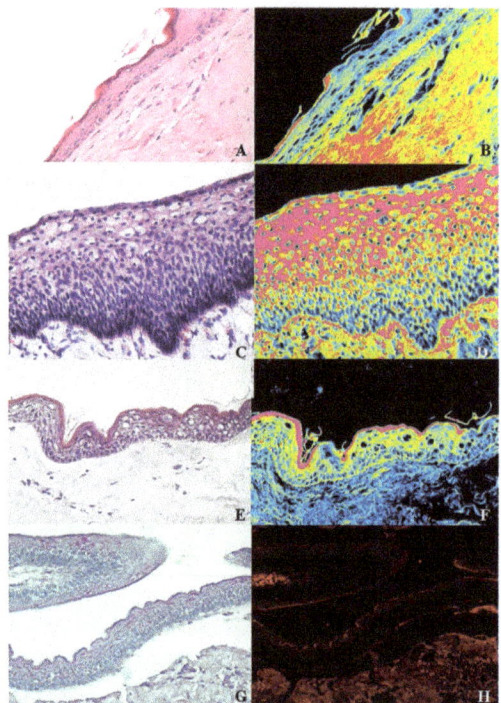

Figure 1. (**A**,**B**) Morphologic appearance of the epithelium in sporadic KOTs with traditional microscopy (haematoxylin–eosin staining) and the same field in Confocal Laser Scanning Microscopy with a double laser inducing fluorescence (green and red) (original magnification of ×20). (**C**,**D**) Higher cellular density with subepithelial basophilic layers of syndromic KOTs in traditional microscopy (haematoxylin–eosin staining) and the same field in Confocal Laser Scanning Microscopy with a double laser inducing fluorescence (green and red) (original magnification of ×20). (**E**,**F**) Low cellular density without subepithelial basophilic layers of sporadic KOTs in traditional microscopy (haematoxylin–eosin staining) and the same field in Confocal Laser Scanning Microscopy with a double laser inducing fluorescence (green and red) (original magnification of ×20). (**G**,**H**) Epithelial detachment in syndromic KOTs due to the amorphous and fragile basement membrane in traditional microscopy (haematoxylin–eosin staining) and the same field in Confocal Laser Scanning Microscopy with a red laser inducing fluorescence (original magnification of ×20).

Table 2. CLSM typical features of 120 syndromic and 93 sporadic OKs.

	Syndromic OKs	Non-Syndromic OKs
Satellite cysts	+++	+
Subepithelial basophilic layers	+	-
Cellular density	+++	+
Basement membrane	Fragile	Resistant
Epithelial lining	Epithelial detachment and scalloped aspect	Lack of epithelial detachment

+++: numerous. +: detectable. -: absent.

4. Discussion

Following its initial designation as a cyst of odontogenic origin, some authors postulated that OKs would have been more appropriately considered neoplasms, in view of their locally destructive and aggressive behaviour, high recurrence rates after simple enucleation, histological appearance, expression of tumour markers, and for the occurrence of the mutation of the PTCH1 gene [2,3,9,14]. Such tentative re-classification of OKs as neoplastic lesions (keratocystic odontogenic tumour) was included in the WHO classifications of 2005 of odontogenic tumours to highlight its virtually aggressive nature and to emphasize the need for more aggressive therapeutic interventions [18]. Nevertheless, no unanimous consensus was reached in this regard, and in the updated WHO classifications, OKs were re-included among the odontogenic cysts, with a note of caution as to its possible aggressive behaviour [4–6].

In close agreement with most reports in the literature, the mean age of NBCCS patients in the current series was lower than that of patients harbouring non-syndromic OKs; the male–female ratio was almost 1.5:1, thus confirming the slight male predominance generally reported by several investigators [2]. Most reports concur that OKs affect the mandible more frequently than the maxilla, with the mandibular posterior region being the most commonly affected site, as confirmed by our analyses, which also support the prevalence of mandibular OKs in sporadic lesions.

While we detected a relatively smaller percentage (20.19%) of OKs associated with impacted teeth than what reported in the literature [19], our data confirm that multiple OKs were mostly detected within NBCCS patients, who also experienced higher recurrence rates and larger sizes of the lesions. Quite interestingly, the recurrence rate of OKs in non-syndromic patients included in the current series was lower than the one reported in the literature, with analogous treatment modalities [19–22].

Biological differences between sporadic and syndromic keratocysts were studied performing an immunohistochemical evaluation of the Sonic-Hedgehog-signalling-pathway protein expression (Shh, Ptch1, Ptch2, Smo, Gli1, Gli2, and Gli3), and it emerged that in the syndromic OKs, there was an increase in the expression of Shh, Smo, and Gli1 proteins when compared to that of sporadic cysts [23].

Some novel findings of this study resulted from the CLSM examination of the histological samples using autofluorescence. CLSM was demonstrated to be a major advance in biological imaging and in many fields of dental medicine [24,25], as well as in general medicine [25,26]. It may be considered an intermediate step between optical and electronic microscopy and uses a bi-chromatic punctiform laser source, the resulting emission energy being detected by a spatially filtered optical system, the pinhole, which eliminates light signals arising from out-of-focus planes [24]. Samples do not need any specific staining procedure, as conventional H&E-stained sections provide excellent results. Overall, CLSM produces intensely stained and high-resolution images, with clearly visible borders, without noise or otherwise disturbing signals from the surrounding tissues.

In the current study, CLSM allowed us to perform more accurate analyses of the morphological and cellular features of the lesions, in particular, the detection of amorphous and fragile basement membranes, detached and collapsed epithelial layers, and higher cellular density in the basal epithelial layers with increased proliferative activity in syndromic OKs as compared with sporadic lesions. Such features may at least in part justify the higher tendency of syndromic OKs to recur, in view of the lower mechanical resistance of the peripheral layers of the cysts towards the expansion of the proliferating epithelial compartment.

Our study has limitations, such as the lack of discrimination between orthokeratinized and parakeratinized keratocysts and the absence of a correlation with an immunohistochemical analysis.

In addition, considering CLSM as a quick and easily manageable technique in oral pathology, it may be adopted as a supplementary tool, along with immunohistochemistry and molecular biology, to tell apart syndromic from sporadic OKs, especially in cases in which the surgical samples may result insufficient for extensive morphologic evaluation [27,28].

Author Contributions: Conceptualization, G.F. and L.L.; methodology, G.F. and E.M.; software, E.M.; validation, F.S. and A.T.; formal analysis, S.C.; investigation, E.M.; resources, A.T.; data curation, L.L.; writing—original draft preparation, G.F.; writing—review and editing, F.S. and L.L.M.; visualization, E.L.M.; supervision, L.L.M. All authors have read and agreed to the published version of the manuscript.

Funding: This research study received no external funding.

Institutional Review Board Statement: The study was conducted in accordance with the Declaration of Helsinki and approved by the institutional review board (study No. 4599, Prot. 1528/C.E).

Informed Consent Statement: Informed consent was obtained from all subjects involved in the study.

Data Availability Statement: Not applicable.

Acknowledgments: This work was supported by Consorzio Interuniversitario Nazionale per la Bio-Oncologia (CINBO), Italy.

Conflicts of Interest: The authors declare no conflict of interest.

References

1. Philipsen, H.P. Om keratocystedr (Kolesteratomer) and kaeberne. *Tandlaegebladet* **1956**, *60*, 963–971.
2. Bhargava, D.; Deshpande, A.; Pogrel, M.A. Keratocystic odontogenic tumour (KCOT)-a cyst to a tumour. *Oral Maxillofac. Surg.* **2012**, *16*, 163–170. [CrossRef] [PubMed]
3. Barnes, L.; Eveson, J.W.; Reichart, P.; Sidransky, D. *Pathology and Genetics of Head and Neck Tumours*; IARC Press: Lyon, France, 2005.
4. Speight, P.; Devilliers, P.; Li, T.-J.; Odell, E.W.; Wright, J.M. Odontogenic keratocyst. In *WHO Classification of Head and Neck Tumours*, 4th ed.; El-Naggar, A.K., Chan, J.K.C., Grandis, J.R., Takata, T., Slootweg, P., Eds.; IARC Press: Lyon, France, 2017.
5. Bhargava, D. Odontogenic keratocyst (OKC)-reverting back from tumour to cyst: Keratocystic odontogenic tumour (KCOT)-a cyst to a tumour. *Oral Maxillofac. Surg.* **2012**, *16*, 163–170. [CrossRef] [PubMed]
6. Vered, M.; Wright, J.M. Update from the 5th Edition of the World Health Organization Classification of Head and Neck Tumors: Odontogenic and Maxillofacial Bone Tumours. *Head Neck Pathol.* **2022**, *16*, 63–75. [CrossRef]
7. Gorlin, R.J.; Goltz, R.W. Multiple nevoid basal-cell epithelioma, jaw cysts and bifid rib. A syndrome. *N. Engl. J. Med.* **1960**, *262*, 908–912. [CrossRef]
8. Soluk-Tekkesin, M.; Wright, J.M. The World Health Organization Classification of Odontogenic Lesions: A Summary of the Changes of the 2022 (5th) Edition. *Turk. Patoloji. Derg.* **2022**, *38*, 168–184. [CrossRef]
9. Pogrel, M.A. The keratocystic odontogenic tumor. *Oral Maxillofac. Surg. Clin. N. Am.* **2013**, *25*, 21–30. [CrossRef]
10. Stoelinga, P.J. Etiology and pathogenesis of keratocysts. *Oral Maxillofac. Surg. Clin. N. Am.* **2003**, *15*, 317–324. [CrossRef]
11. Gorlin, R.J. Nevoid basal cell carcinoma syndrome. *Dermatol. Clin.* **1995**, *13*, 113–125. [CrossRef]
12. Eryilmaz, T.; Ozmen, S.; Findikcioglu, K.; Kandal, S.; Aral, M. Odontogenic keratocyst: An unusual location and review of the literature. *Ann. Plast. Surg.* **2009**, *62*, 210–212. [CrossRef]
13. Stoelinga, P.J. Long-term follow-up on keratocysts treated according to a defined protocol. *Int. J. Oral Maxillofac. Surg.* **2001**, *30*, 14–25. [CrossRef] [PubMed]
14. Abdullah, W.A. Surgical treatment of keratocystic odontogenic tumour: A review article. *Saudi Dent. J.* **2011**, *23*, 61–65. [CrossRef] [PubMed]
15. Ravi, J.; Wadhwan, V.; Gotur, S.P. Orthokeratinized versus parakeratinized odontogenic keratocyst: Our institutional experience. *J. Oral. Maxillofac. Pathol.* **2022**, *26*, 60–64. [CrossRef] [PubMed]

16. Selvamani, M.; Devi, A.Y.; Basandi, P.S.; Madhushankari, G.S. Prevalence and clinicopathological comparison of kerotocystic odontogenic tumor and orthokeratinized odontogenic cyst in South Indian sample population: A retrospective study over 13 years. *J. Pharm. Bioallied. Sci.* **2014**, *6*, S127–S130. [CrossRef]
17. Betancourt, N.J.; Qian, M.F.; Pickford, J.R.; Bailey-Healy, I.; Tang, J.Y.; Teng, J.M.C. Gorlin Syndrome: Assessing Genotype-Phenotype Correlations and Analysis of Early Clinical Characteristics as Risk Factors for Disease Severity. *J. Clin. Oncol.* **2022**, *40*, 2119–2127. [CrossRef]
18. Madras, J.; Lapointe, H. Keratocystic odontogenic tumour: Reclassification of the odontogenic keratocyst from cyst to tumour. *J. Can. Dent. Assoc.* **2008**, *74*, 165.
19. Chirapathomsakul, D.; Sastravaha, P.; Jansisyanont, P. A review of odontogenic keratocysts and the behavior of recurrences. *Oral Surg. Oral Med. Oral Pathol. Oral Radiol. Endod.* **2006**, *101*, 5–9. [CrossRef]
20. Bataineh, A.B.; al Qudah, M. Treatment of mandibular odontogenic keratocysts. *Oral Surg. Oral Med. Oral Pathol. Oral Radiol. Endod.* **1998**, *86*, 42–47. [CrossRef]
21. Driemel, O.; Rieder, J.; Morsczeck, C.; Schwarz, S.; Hakim, S.G.; Muller-Richter, U.; Reichert, T.E.; Kosmehl, H. Comparison of clinical immunohistochemical findings in keratocystic odontogenic tumours and ameloblastomas considering their risk of recurrence. *Mund-Kiefer-Gesichtschirurgie MKG* **2007**, *11*, 221–231. [CrossRef]
22. Habibi, A.; Saghravanian, N.; Habibi, M.; Mellati, E.; Habibi, M. Keratocystic odontogenic tumor: A 10-year retrospective study of 83 cases in an Iranian population. *J. Oral Sci.* **2007**, *49*, 229–235. [CrossRef]
23. Hoyos Cadavid, A.M.; Kaminagakura, E.; Rodrigues, M.; Pinto, C.A.L.; Teshima, T.H.N.; Alves, F.A. Immunohistochemical evaluation of Sonic Hedgehog signaling pathway proteins (Shh, Ptch1, Ptch2, Smo, Gli1, Gli2, and Gli3) in sporadic and syndromic odontogenic keratocysts. *Clin. Oral. Investig.* **2019**, *23*, 153–159. [CrossRef] [PubMed]
24. Zucker, R.M.; Price, O. Evaluation of confocal microscopy system performance. *Cytometry* **2001**, *44*, 273–294. [CrossRef]
25. Watson, T.F. Applications of confocal scanning optical microscopy to dentistry. *Br. Dent. J.* **1991**, *171*, 287–291. [CrossRef] [PubMed]
26. Zucker, R.M.; Price, O.T. Practical confocal microscopy and the evaluation of system performance. *Methods* **1999**, *18*, 447–458. [CrossRef] [PubMed]
27. Cserni, D.; Zombori, T.; Stajer, A.; Rimovszki, A.; Cserni, G.; Barath, Z. Immunohistochemical Characterization of Reactive Epithelial Changes in Odontogenic Keratocysts. *Pathol. Oncol. Res.* **2020**, *26*, 1717–1724. [CrossRef]
28. Vered, M.; Peleg, O.; Taicher, S.; Buchner, A. The immunoprofile of odontogenic keratocyst (keratocystic odontogenic tumor) that includes expression of PTCH, SMO, GLI-1 and bcl-2 is similar to ameloblastoma but different from odontogenic cysts. *J. Oral Pathol. Med.* **2009**, *38*, 597–604. [CrossRef]

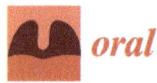

Review

Intraoral Sialadenoma Papilliferum: A Comprehensive Review of the Literature with Emphasis on Clinical and Histopathological Diagnostic Features

Rita Antonelli [1], Oslei Paes de Almeida [2], Ronell Bologna-Molina [3] and Marco Meleti [1,*]

[1] Centro Universitario Odontoiatria, Department of Medicine and Surgery, University of Parma, 43126 Parma, Italy
[2] Oral Diagnosis Department, Oral Pathology Section, Piracicaba Dental School, University of Campinas (UNICAMP), Piracicaba 1314-903, Sao Paolo, Brazil
[3] Molecular Pathology Area, School of Dentistry, Universidad de la República (UDELAR), Montevideo 14600, Uruguay
* Correspondence: marco.meleti@unipr.it

Abstract: Background. Sialadenoma papilliferum (SP) is a rare benign epithelial tumor of salivary gland origin, its diagnosis being potentially challenging. It was first described by Abrams and Finck in 1969 as an analog of the cutaneous syringocystadenoma papilliferum. The aim of this comprehensive review is to highlight the clinical and histopathological diagnostic aspects of intraoral SP, analyzing cases previously described and reporting new cases. Methods. Medline, Scopus, and Web of Science were searched up to February 2022, using as entry term "sialadenoma papilliferum". No time limits were applied and only studies in English were taken into account. Only cases involving the mouth were included. Conference proceedings, personal communications, and letters to the editor were excluded. Results. In total, 42 out of 234 articles fulfilled the inclusion criteria, with 64 cases reported. Mean age of patients with SP was 57.2 years, with a higher prevalence among males. The most affected site was the palate, particularly the hard palate. Four cases with uncertain malignant features have been reported. While clinical manifestations of SP are rather unspecific (e.g., submucosal swelling with ulceration), histopathological and immunohistochemical features are quite peculiar, SP have a limited growth potential, leading to conservative excision as treatment of choice. Conclusions. SP, though rare, should be taken into consideration in the differential diagnosis of intraoral swellings, particularly those located on the palate.

Keywords: sialadenoma papilliferum; salivary gland tumors; oral pathology; oral medicine; oral surgery

Citation: Antonelli, R.; Paes de Almeida, O.; Bologna-Molina, R.; Meleti, M. Intraoral Sialadenoma Papilliferum: A Comprehensive Review of the Literature with Emphasis on Clinical and Histopathological Diagnostic Features. *Oral* **2022**, *2*, 242–250. https://doi.org/10.3390/oral2030023

Academic Editor: Keiichi Tsukinoki

Received: 17 August 2022
Accepted: 6 September 2022
Published: 16 September 2022

Publisher's Note: MDPI stays neutral with regard to jurisdictional claims in published maps and institutional affiliations.

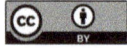

Copyright: © 2022 by the authors. Licensee MDPI, Basel, Switzerland. This article is an open access article distributed under the terms and conditions of the Creative Commons Attribution (CC BY) license (https:// creativecommons.org/licenses/by/ 4.0/).

1. Introduction

Benign and malignant intraoral salivary gland tumors may originate from minor and sublingual salivary glands, as well as from Stensen's and Wharton's ducts. Among benign lesions, sialadenoma papilliferum (SP) is exceedingly rare; its diagnosis being potentially challenging [1]. In the last World Health Organization (WHO) classification of salivary gland tumors, SP has been included in the group of benign epithelial tumors [2].

SP was first documented by Abrams and Finck in 1969 [1], and only 63 intraoral cases have been reported in the English literature since then. According to Waldrom et al., SP accounts for 1.1% of minor salivary gland tumors and for 2% of benign tumors of these glands [3].

The origin of the name lays on the histopathological similarity with syringocystadenoma papilliferum, an uncommon benign tumor of sweat glands origin that has a predilection for the scalp and forehead [4].

Here, we report a comprehensive review of the literature, emphasizing the clinical and histopathological aspects of intraoral SP.

16. Selvamani, M.; Devi, A.Y.; Basandi, P.S.; Madhushankari, G.S. Prevalence and clinicopathological comparison of kerotocystic odontogenic tumor and orthokeratinized odontogenic cyst in South Indian sample population: A retrospective study over 13 years. *J. Pharm. Bioallied. Sci.* **2014**, *6*, S127–S130. [CrossRef]
17. Betancourt, N.J.; Qian, M.F.; Pickford, J.R.; Bailey-Healy, I.; Tang, J.Y.; Teng, J.M.C. Gorlin Syndrome: Assessing Genotype-Phenotype Correlations and Analysis of Early Clinical Characteristics as Risk Factors for Disease Severity. *J. Clin. Oncol.* **2022**, *40*, 2119–2127. [CrossRef]
18. Madras, J.; Lapointe, H. Keratocystic odontogenic tumour: Reclassification of the odontogenic keratocyst from cyst to tumour. *J. Can. Dent. Assoc.* **2008**, *74*, 165.
19. Chirapathomsakul, D.; Sastravaha, P.; Jansisyanont, P. A review of odontogenic keratocysts and the behavior of recurrences. *Oral Surg. Oral Med. Oral Pathol. Oral Radiol. Endod.* **2006**, *101*, 5–9. [CrossRef]
20. Bataineh, A.B.; al Qudah, M. Treatment of mandibular odontogenic keratocysts. *Oral Surg. Oral Med. Oral Pathol. Oral Radiol. Endod.* **1998**, *86*, 42–47. [CrossRef]
21. Driemel, O.; Rieder, J.; Morsczeck, C.; Schwarz, S.; Hakim, S.G.; Muller-Richter, U.; Reichert, T.E.; Kosmehl, H. Comparison of clinical immunohistochemical findings in keratocystic odontogenic tumours and ameloblastomas considering their risk of recurrence. *Mund-Kiefer-Gesichtschirurgie MKG* **2007**, *11*, 221–231. [CrossRef]
22. Habibi, A.; Saghravanian, N.; Habibi, M.; Mellati, E.; Habibi, M. Keratocystic odontogenic tumor: A 10-year retrospective study of 83 cases in an Iranian population. *J. Oral Sci.* **2007**, *49*, 229–235. [CrossRef]
23. Hoyos Cadavid, A.M.; Kaminagakura, E.; Rodrigues, M.; Pinto, C.A.L.; Teshima, T.H.N.; Alves, F.A. Immunohistochemical evaluation of Sonic Hedgehog signaling pathway proteins (Shh, Ptch1, Ptch2, Smo, Gli1, Gli2, and Gli3) in sporadic and syndromic odontogenic keratocysts. *Clin. Oral. Investig.* **2019**, *23*, 153–159. [CrossRef] [PubMed]
24. Zucker, R.M.; Price, O. Evaluation of confocal microscopy system performance. *Cytometry* **2001**, *44*, 273–294. [CrossRef]
25. Watson, T.F. Applications of confocal scanning optical microscopy to dentistry. *Br. Dent. J.* **1991**, *171*, 287–291. [CrossRef] [PubMed]
26. Zucker, R.M.; Price, O.T. Practical confocal microscopy and the evaluation of system performance. *Methods* **1999**, *18*, 447–458. [CrossRef] [PubMed]
27. Cserni, D.; Zombori, T.; Stajer, A.; Rimovszki, A.; Cserni, G.; Barath, Z. Immunohistochemical Characterization of Reactive Epithelial Changes in Odontogenic Keratocysts. *Pathol. Oncol. Res.* **2020**, *26*, 1717–1724. [CrossRef]
28. Vered, M.; Peleg, O.; Taicher, S.; Buchner, A. The immunoprofile of odontogenic keratocyst (keratocystic odontogenic tumor) that includes expression of PTCH, SMO, GLI-1 and bcl-2 is similar to ameloblastoma but different from odontogenic cysts. *J. Oral Pathol. Med.* **2009**, *38*, 597–604. [CrossRef]

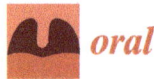

Review

Intraoral Sialadenoma Papilliferum: A Comprehensive Review of the Literature with Emphasis on Clinical and Histopathological Diagnostic Features

Rita Antonelli [1], Oslei Paes de Almeida [2], Ronell Bologna-Molina [3] and Marco Meleti [1,*]

1. Centro Universitario Odontoiatria, Department of Medicine and Surgery, University of Parma, 43126 Parma, Italy
2. Oral Diagnosis Department, Oral Pathology Section, Piracicaba Dental School, University of Campinas (UNICAMP), Piracicaba 1314-903, Sao Paolo, Brazil
3. Molecular Pathology Area, School of Dentistry, Universidad de la República (UDELAR), Montevideo 14600, Uruguay
* Correspondence: marco.meleti@unipr.it

Citation: Antonelli, R.; Paes de Almeida, O.; Bologna-Molina, R.; Meleti, M. Intraoral Sialadenoma Papilliferum: A Comprehensive Review of the Literature with Emphasis on Clinical and Histopathological Diagnostic Features. *Oral* **2022**, *2*, 242–250. https://doi.org/10.3390/oral2030023

Academic Editor: Keiichi Tsukinoki

Received: 17 August 2022
Accepted: 6 September 2022
Published: 16 September 2022

Publisher's Note: MDPI stays neutral with regard to jurisdictional claims in published maps and institutional affiliations.

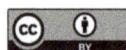

Copyright: © 2022 by the authors. Licensee MDPI, Basel, Switzerland. This article is an open access article distributed under the terms and conditions of the Creative Commons Attribution (CC BY) license (https://creativecommons.org/licenses/by/4.0/).

Abstract: Background. Sialadenoma papilliferum (SP) is a rare benign epithelial tumor of salivary gland origin, its diagnosis being potentially challenging. It was first described by Abrams and Finck in 1969 as an analog of the cutaneous syringocystadenoma papilliferum. The aim of this comprehensive review is to highlight the clinical and histopathological diagnostic aspects of intraoral SP, analyzing cases previously described and reporting new cases. Methods. Medline, Scopus, and Web of Science were searched up to February 2022, using as entry term "sialadenoma papilliferum". No time limits were applied and only studies in English were taken into account. Only cases involving the mouth were included. Conference proceedings, personal communications, and letters to the editor were excluded. Results. In total, 42 out of 234 articles fulfilled the inclusion criteria, with 64 cases reported. Mean age of patients with SP was 57.2 years, with a higher prevalence among males. The most affected site was the palate, particularly the hard palate. Four cases with uncertain malignant features have been reported. While clinical manifestations of SP are rather unspecific (e.g., submucosal swelling with ulceration), histopathological and immunohistochemical features are quite peculiar, SP have a limited growth potential, leading to conservative excision as treatment of choice. Conclusions. SP, though rare, should be taken into consideration in the differential diagnosis of intraoral swellings, particularly those located on the palate.

Keywords: sialadenoma papilliferum; salivary gland tumors; oral pathology; oral medicine; oral surgery

1. Introduction

Benign and malignant intraoral salivary gland tumors may originate from minor and sublingual salivary glands, as well as from Stensen's and Wharton's ducts. Among benign lesions, sialadenoma papilliferum (SP) is exceedingly rare; its diagnosis being potentially challenging [1]. In the last World Health Organization (WHO) classification of salivary gland tumors, SP has been included in the group of benign epithelial tumors [2].

SP was first documented by Abrams and Finck in 1969 [1], and only 63 intraoral cases have been reported in the English literature since then. According to Waldrom et al., SP accounts for 1.1% of minor salivary gland tumors and for 2% of benign tumors of these glands [3].

The origin of the name lays on the histopathological similarity with syringocystadenoma papilliferum, an uncommon benign tumor of sweat glands origin that has a predilection for the scalp and forehead [4].

Here, we report a comprehensive review of the literature, emphasizing the clinical and histopathological aspects of intraoral SP.

2. Materials and Methods

The Medline, Scopus, and Web of Science databases were searched using as entry term "sialadenoma papilliferum".

Database screening was performed until February 2022. No time limits were applied and only studies in English were considered. Only cases involving the mouth were included. Conference proceedings, personal communications, and letters to the editor were excluded.

First level screening was performed on titles and/or abstracts, and full-text was evaluated in controversial cases. References lists in reviews were screened in order to identify papers possibly missing from the databases search.

Information extracted included title, authors, year of publication, number of reported cases, oral subsite, and size of lesions (Table 1).

Table 1. Data of the 42 articles (64 cases) included in the present review.

Title	Authors	Year	n° Cases Reported	Age, Sex	Oral Subsite	Size of Lesions (cm)
Sialoadenoma papilliferum. A Previously Unreported Salivary Gland Tumor [1]	Abrams, A.M. and Finck, F.M.	1969	1	57, M	Hard and soft right palate junction	1.5
Sialoadenoma papilliferum: report of case [5]	Crocker, D.J., et al.	1972	1	71, M	Left buccal mucosa	0.6
SialadenomaPapillifemm of the Oral Cavity [6]	Jensen, J.L. and Reingold, I.M.	1973	1	48, M	Hard palate	0.8
Papillary tumors of the minor salivary glands [7]	Whittaker, J.P. and Mer, E.E.	1976	2	50, M	Hard and soft palate junction	0.6
				65, M	Hard palate	N/A
Sialoadenoma papilliferum of the oral cavity [8]	Drummond, J.F., et al.	1978	1	71, M	Left mandibular retromolar area	0.5
Sialoadenoma papilliferum [9]	Freedman, P.D. and Lumerman, H.	1978	2	68, M	Hard palate lateral to the midline	0.3
				68, M	Left hard palate	0.5
Intraoral papillary squamous cell tumor of the soft palate with features of sialoadenoma papilliferum? Malignant sialoadenoma papilliferum [10]	Solomon, M.P., et al.	1978	1	62, M	Soft palate	4.0
Sialoadenoma papilliferum [11]	Mccoy, J.M. and Eckert, J.R.E.F.	1980	1	77, F	Right buccal mucosa	0.7
Sialoadenoma papilliferum. Report of a case [12]	Nasu, M., et al.	1981	1	61, M	Hard palate	0.6
Sialoadenoma papilliferum [13]	Wertheimer, F.W., et al.	1983	2	32, F	Hard palate	0.4
				43, M	Soft palate	0.5
Sialocystadenoma papilliferum of the palate [14]	Puts, J.J., et al.	1984	1	71, M	Hard palate	1.6
Sialadenoma papilliferum. A case report and review of the literature [15]	Rennie, J.S., et al.	1984	1	78, F	Hard and soft palate junction	1.0
Ultrastructure of a sialoadenoma papilliferum [16]	Kanemitsu, S., et al.	1984	1	58, M	Hard palate	0.7
Sialoadenoma papilliferum [17]	Bass, K.D. and Cosentino, B.J.	1985	1	76, F	Left faucial pillar	1.0
Minor salivary gland tumors. A histologic and immunohisto chemical study [18]	Regezi, J.A., et al.	1985	2	63, M	Hard palate	N/A
				79, F	Hard palate	N/A
Ultrastructure of sialoadenoma papilliferum [19]	Fantasia, J.E., et al.	1986	5	87, F	Hard palate	N/A
				77, M	Buccal mucosa	N/A
				48, F	Hard palate	N/A
				45, M	Hard palate	N/A
				60, F	Mucosa upper lip	N/A
Sialoadenoma papilliferum: report of case and review of literature [20]	Mitre, B.K.	1986	1	42, F	Hard and soft palate junction	0.4
Sialoadenoma papilliferum of the oral cavity: a case report and review of the literature [21]	Papanicolaou, S. and Triantafyllou, A.G.	1987	1	46, M	Hard palate	0.5
The rare sialoadenoma papilliferum—report of a case and review of the literature [22]	Van der Wal, J.E. and van der Waal, I.	1991	1	46, M	Hard and soft palate junction	0.5
Recurrent sialadenoma papilliferum of the buccal mucosa [23]	Pimentel, M.T.Y., et al.	1995	1	65, F	Buccal mucosa	2.0
Sialadenoma papilliferum: an immunohistochemical study of five cases [24]	Maiorano, E., et al.	1996	5	56, M	Hard palate	0.5
				37, F	Hard palate	1.0
				60, M	Cheek	0.8
				46, M	Hard palate	1.4
				50, M	Hard palate	1.8

Table 1. Cont.

Title	Authors	Year	n° Cases Reported	Age, Sex	Oral Subsite	Size of Lesions (cm)
Sialadenoma papilliferum of the oral cavity: report of a case and literature review [25]	Markopoulos, A., et al.	1997	1	50, M	Hard palate	0.5
Sialadenoma papilliferum of the hard palate: a case report of a case and review of literature [26]	Asahina, I. and Masato, A.	1997	1	50, M	Hard palate	0.4
Sialadenoma papilliferum of the palate: case report and literature review [27]	Argyres, M.I. and Golitz, L.E.	1998	1	50, M	Hard palate	0.5
Ductal papillomas of salivary gland origin: A report of 19 cases and a review of the literature [28]	Brannon, R.B., et al.	2001	3	69, F 53, F 31, F	Hard palate Soft palate Hard palate	N/A N/A N/A
Sialadenoma papilliferum of the hard palate—Report of 2 cases and immunohistochemical evaluation [29]	Ubaidat, M.A., et al.	2001	2	72, M 58, M	Hard palate Hard palate	0.4 0.5
Malignant transformation of sialadenoma papilliferum of the palate: a case report [30]	Shimoda, M., et al.	2004	1	79, F	Hard and soft palate junction	4.0
Sialadenoma papilliferum: Immunohistochemical study [31]	Gomes, A.P.N., et al.	2004	2	53, M 52, F	Hard palate Soft palate	1.0 0.5
Sialadenoma papilliferum in a young patient: a case report and review of the literature [32]	Mahajan, D., et al.	2007	1	18, M	Upper lip	0.8
A rare case of sialadenoma papilliferum with epithelial dysplasia and carcinoma in situ [33]	Ponniah, I.	2007	1	30, M	Floor of the mouth	1.5
Minor salivary gland tumors: A clinicopathological study of 18 cases [34]	Vicente, O.P., et al.	2008	1	46, F	Hard palate	N/A
Mucoepidermoid carcinoma arising in a background of sialadenoma papilliferum: A case report [35]	Liu, W., et al.	2009	1	82, F	Left base of the tongue	N/A
Sialadenoma papilliferum with potentially malignant features [36]	Ide, F., et al.	2010	1	67, M	Right retromolar alveolar ridge	3.0
Sialadenoma papilliferum of the hard palate: A case report [37]	Kubota, Y., et al.	2012	1	62, M	Hard palate	1.0
Sialadenoma papilliferum: clinical misdiagnosis with a histological decree [38]	Anuradha, A., et al.	2012	1	65, M	Floor of the mouth	1.0
Sialadenoma Papilliferum with inverted pattern in a young patient: a case report [39]	Reis de Sá Silva e Costa, F.E., et al.	2015	1	20, M	Upper lip buccal mucosa	1.3
Sialadenoma papilliferum of the tongue mimicking a malignant tumor [40]	Santos, J.N., et al.	2013	1	32, F	Posteriore lateral border of the tongue	1.0
Sialadenoma Papilliferum: Analysis of Seven New Cases and Review of the Literature [41]	Fowler, C.B. and Damm, D.D.	2017	7	55, F 50, M 62, M 63, M 57, M 48, F 76, F	Hard palate Hard palate Hard palate Hard palate Palate Hard palate Hard palate	0.3 0.8 N/A N/A 0.4 0.5 1.3
Sialadenoma papilliferum in the buccal mucosa detected on (18)F-fluorodeoxyglucose-positron emission tomography [42]	Miyamoto, S., et al.	2017	1	53, M	Left buccal mucosa	0.8
Sialadenoma papilliferum: A rare case report and review of literature [43]	Sunil, S., et al.	2017	1	58, F	Hard palate	1.0
Sialadenoma papilliferum of the hard palate: A rare case report [44]	Atarbashi-Moghadam, S., et al.	2019	1	50, F	Hard palate	1.0
Sialadenoma papilliferum: Special staining and immunohistochemical staining [45]	Takasugi, N., et al.	2021	1	83, F	Hard palate	0.8

N/A = information not available.

Search flow is summarized in Scheme 1.

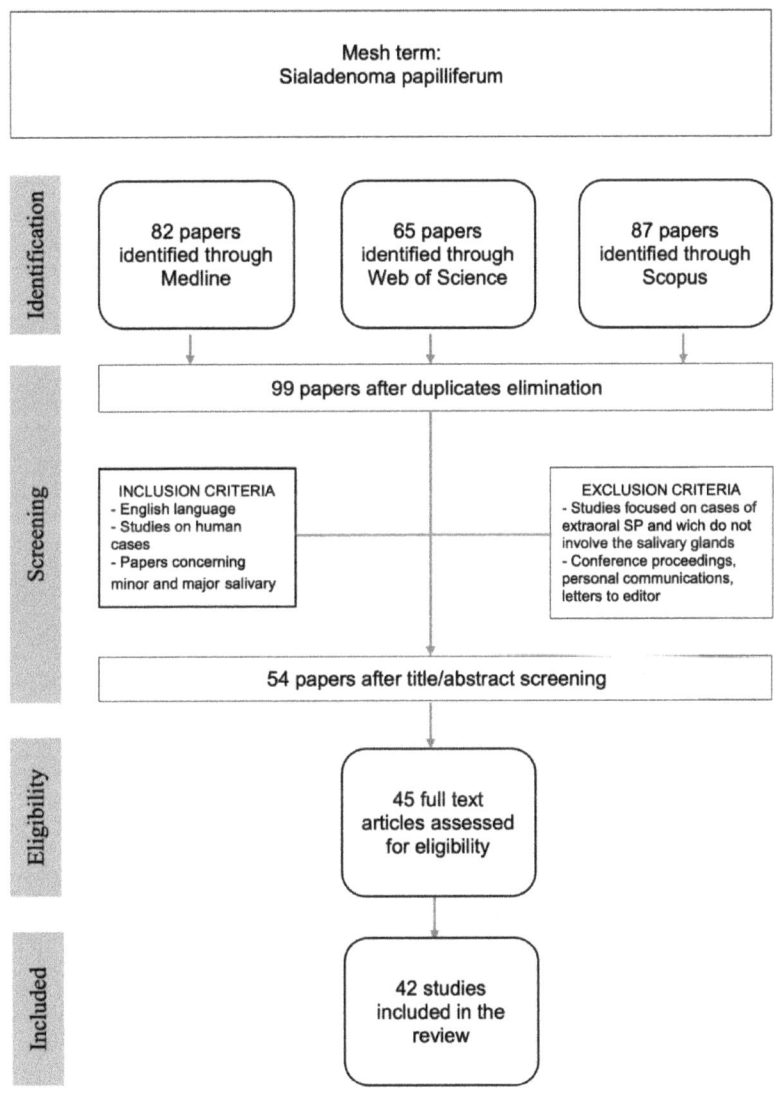

Scheme 1. Flow chart diagram for the selection of 42 papers included in the review.

3. Results

Databases search returned a list of 234 papers which were reduced to 99 after the elimination of duplicates. After abstract and full-text evaluation, 42 articles qualified as specifically reporting on SP of the mouth and were therefore included for further data extrapolation and analysis. Only to mention that 4 cases of SP affecting the parotid were found that according to the criteria used were excluded [1,46–48].

Eventually, 64 cases were identified since Abrams' and Finck's [1] first description of the lesion in 1969 (Table 1).

3.1. Age and Sex

Age ranged from 18 to 87 years, with a mean age of 57.2, all in patients older than 30 years, except 2 cases affecting a male of 18 years and a male of 20 years.

The present review has highlighted a predominance of SP among males (39 males, 25 females; M/F ratio: 1.6:1).

3.2. Clinical Features

The palate was the most common involved site, with 48 (75%) cases, of these specifically, 37 (58%) were on the hard palate, 6 (9.5%) on the hard and soft palate junction, 4 (6%) on the soft palate and 1 (1.5%) on unspecified palatal localization.

Other sites included buccal mucosa (6; 9.5%), upper lip mucosa (3; 5%), mandibular retromolar area (2; 3%), floor of the mouth (2; 3%), tongue (2; 3%), and left faucial pillar (1; 1.5%).

SP usually presents as an asymptomatic, a slow growing, and a papillary exophytic lesion. In most cases an erythematous area within an otherwise normal mucosa is present (Figure 1A). Most frequent differential diagnoses is papilloma, on the basis of the keratotic appearance with papillary surface. Other clinical diagnostic hypotheses include palatal fistulas, pyogenic granuloma, soft tissues neoplasms and other benign and malignant minor salivary gland tumors.

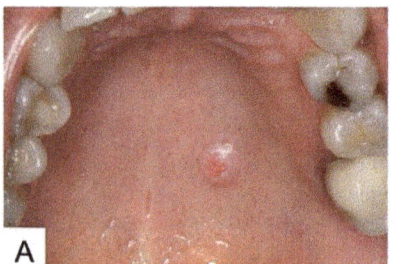
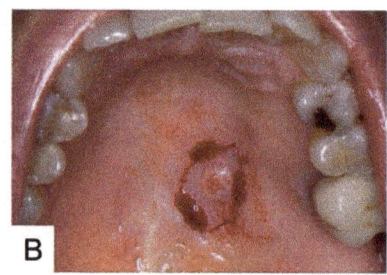
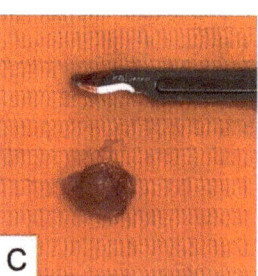

Figure 1. (**A**) Sialoadenoma papilliferum on the hard palate of a 48-year-old female patient; (**B**) Surgical excision under local anesthesia; (**C**) Surgical specimen.

In the cases analyzed in the present review, tumor size ranged from very small (0.3 cm) to large lesions up to 4 cm, with a mean size of 0.79 cm.

Larger cases up to 7 cm can occur in the parotid and again up to now with four cases described including Abram's case [1,46].

3.3. Histological Features

Histological description of cases evaluated in the present analysis were very similar, the histopathologic pattern of SP being rather characteristic.

The tumor seems to originate from the superficial portion of salivary glands excretory ducts. Papillary processes develop, eventually forming convoluted cleft and spaces. Each papillary projection is lined by consisting of two or three layers of cells, supported by a core of fibrovascular connective tissue. The most superficial portions of the lesion have a squamous epithelial lining; deeper areas show mainly cuboidal to columnar cells, often oncocytic in appearance (Figure 2). As growth progresses, the overlying mucous membrane becomes papillary or verrucous, much like a squamous papilloma.

Various research has attempted to identify the cell of origin of SP based on light microscopy, immunohistochemistry (IHC), and electron microscopy (EM) [41]. These methods have yielded variable results with most investigators suggesting excretory duct or excretory duct reserve cell origin [9–12,19,24,29,31,41,44]. Other authors hypothesized an origin from intercalated duct cells [12,49] or myoepithelial cells [1,29,41].

Fowler and Damm documented that basal cell on the ductal structures were immunoreactive for p63 and p40, a myoepithelial immunophenotype [41]. Variable reactivity in the basal cell layer with smooth muscle actin (SMA) was also identified. In all cases reported in their paper, the luminal cells within the ductal structures were immunoreactive to epithelial membrane antigen (EMA). These results indicate two cell types comprising the convoluted ductal structures of SP: a basal layer of myoepithelial cells (p40+, p63+, and SMA+) and a luminal layer of ductal epithelial cells (EMA+) (Figure 3A,B).

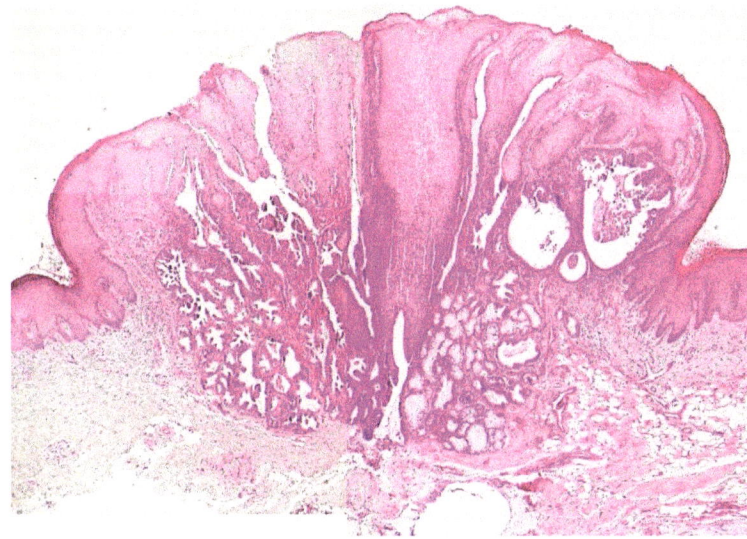

Figure 2. Example of histological features of SP (case different from that presented in Figure 1): exophytic papillary structure covered by stratified squamous epithelium and glandular structures below the mucosa (H&E—50×).

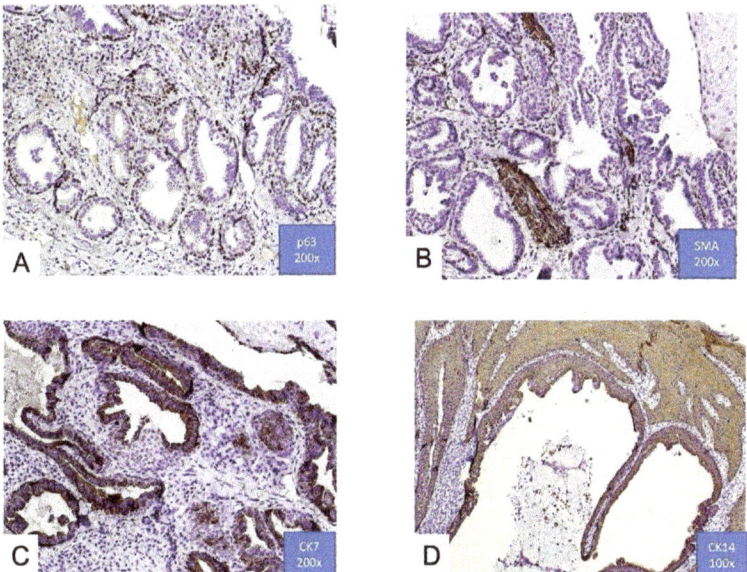

Figure 3. (**A**,**B**) Focal immunohistochemical positivity for p63 and smooth muscle actin (SMA). Immunoreactivity for p63 in basal cells of ductal structures suggesting a myoepithelial immunophenotype. Positivity of ductal structures is also evident; (**C**,**D**) positive immunohistochemical expression for cytokeratins 7 and 14 (CK7 and CK14) in ductal luminal cells, possibly confirming the epithelial origin (100× and 200×).

A recent immunohistochemical analysis reported by Atarbashi-Moghadam et al. shows positivity for cytokeratins 13, 14, 7, 8, and 19, and it is negative for vimentin and smooth muscle actin. This immunoprofile is similar to excretory ducts of the salivary gland [44] (Figure 3C,D).

3.4. Treatment

Conservative excision seems to be the treatment of choice (Figure 1B,C). Because of the rarity of SP, no clinical protocols have been proposed with regard to the possible duration of follow-up. According to van der Wal and van der Waal, follow-up should be scheduled at regular intervals [22].

3.5. Prognosis

SP is a benign neoplasm with limited growth and limited potential for local aggressiveness, recurrence rate is low, with only 2 cases out of 64 described within 3 years after surgical excision [15,23].

3.6. Possible Malignant Transformation

It is uncertain eventual malignant transformation of SP or on the existence of a malignant variant of the tumor. According to this review four cases with uncertain malignancy have been reported.

Solomon et al., presented a case of a possibly malignant SP [10], even though the diagnosis has been challenged by other authors (Ellis, G.L. and Auclair, P.L., 1991).

Ide et al., described an SP with potentially malignant features, such as rapid and destructive growth, radiographic resorption of the underlying bone, and atypical histological features [36].

Santos et al. also reported a case of SP on the tongue with apparently malignant clinical aspects, which led to the clinical diagnosis of squamous cell carcinoma [40].

Shimoda et al. reported the first case of SP with a definite malignant component [30].

However, Fowler and Damm mentioned that there was insufficient evidence to support this diagnosis and to consider that as a malignancy from preexisting SP [41].

In short, whether SP has a malignant potential therefore remains unanswered.

4. Discussion

Salivary gland tumors are a morphologically and clinically diverse group of neoplasms that affect predominantly major salivary glands but also are not uncommon in the minor salivary glands.

The global annual incidence, when all salivary glands tumors are considered, is approximately 1 case per 100,000 per year [49].

Pleomorphic adenoma and mucoepidermoid carcinoma are the two most common benign and malignant minor salivary gland tumors, while SP represents only a small percentage of cases (1.1–1.6%) [3,9].

A usual difficulty in the management of minor salivary gland tumors is the very heterogeneous clinical and radiographic features, as well as the rather wide range of histopathological subtypes.

The exophytic growth pattern of SP is similar to most intraoral salivary gland tumors, which present as submucosal nodular swellings, with or without superficial ulceration. Such a clinic pattern is shared with other lesions, including among others squamous papilloma, verrucous hyperplasia, and exophytic ductal papilloma.

Squamous papilloma and verrucous hyperplasia show only squamous epithelial proliferation and thus can be easily differentiated from SP. Exophytic ductal papilloma displays exophytic papillary ductal epithelial proliferation, but it lacks a ductal proliferation underneath the epithelium. Instead, SP shows as unique histopathologic features an exophytic proliferation of papillary stratified squamous epithelium and a contiguously endophytic salivary ductal proliferation underneath [50].

SP frequently presents as an erythematous lesion, with ulceration or erosion that may suggest a malignant lesion, such as verrucous carcinoma or even sarcomas [38].

From the epidemiological point of view, age and gender are not very helpful in the differential diagnosis, as most salivary gland tumors have no gender predilection and the mean age found in the present review for SP is similar to that reported for other salivary gland tumors (45 years, with a range of 11–74) [51].

SP appears to have a limited growth potential, with an average size at diagnosis of 0.79 cm, facilitating a conservative surgical treatment. There are insufficient data to support the malignant potential of SP, although four cases of supposed malignant transformation were reported.

Research is currently focused to determine the cells of origin of SP, but despite immunohistochemical studies, such question remain unanswered.

In conclusion SP, though rare, should be taken into consideration in the differential diagnosis of intraoral swellings, particularly those located on the palate, and more studies are necessary to better understand its biology.

Author Contributions: Conceptualization, Methodology, Writing—Original Draft Preparation: R.A. Conceptualization, Methodology, Supervision, Writing—Review and Editing: M.M. Writing—Review and Editing: O.P.d.A. and R.B.-M. All authors have read and agreed to the published version of the manuscript.

Funding: This research received no external funding.

Institutional Review Board Statement: Not applicable.

Informed Consent Statement: Not applicable.

Conflicts of Interest: The authors declare no conflict of interest.

References

1. Abrams, A.M.; Finck, F.M. Sialadenoma papilliferum: A previously un-reported salivary gland tumor. *Cancer* **1969**, *24*, 1057–1063. [CrossRef]
2. Seethala, R.R.; Stenman, G. Update from the 4th edition of the world health organization classification of head and neck tumours: Tumors of the salivary gland. *Head Neck Pathol.* **2017**, *11*, 55–67. [CrossRef] [PubMed]
3. Waldron, C.A.; El-Mofty, S.K.; Gnepp, D.R. Tumors of the intraoral minor salivary glands: A demographic and histologic study of 426 cases. *Oral Surg. Oral Med. Oral Pathol.* **1988**, *66*, 323–333. [CrossRef]
4. Seifert, G.; Brocheriou, C.; Cardesa, A.; Eveson, J.W. WHO international classification of tumors. Tentative histological classification of salivary gland tumours. *Pathol. Res. Pract.* **1990**, *186*, 555–581. [CrossRef]
5. Crocker, D.J.; Christ, T.F.; Cavalaris, C.J. Sialadenoma Papilliferum: Report of Case. *J. Oral Surg.* **1972**, *30*, 520–521.
6. Jensen, J.L.; Reingold, I.M. Sialadenoma Papillifemm of the Oral Cavity. *Oral Surg. Oral Med. Oral Pathol.* **1973**, *35*, 521–525. [CrossRef]
7. Whittaker, J.S.; Mer, E.E. Papillary tumors of the minor salivary glands. *J. Clin. Pathol.* **1976**, *29*, 795–805. [CrossRef]
8. Drummond, J.F.; Giansanti, J.S.; Sabes, W.R.; Smith, C.R. Sialadenoma papilliferum of the oral cavity. *Oral Surg. Oral Med. Oral Pathol.* **1978**, *45*, 72–75. [CrossRef]
9. Freedman, P.D.; Lumerman, H. Sialoadenoma papilliferum. *Oral Surg.* **1978**, *45*, 88–94. [CrossRef]
10. Solomon, M.P.; Rosen, Y.; Alfonso, A. Intraoral papillary squamous cell tumor of the soft palate with features of sialadenoma papilliferum? Malignant sialadenoma papilliferum. *Cancer* **1978**, *42*, 1859–1869.
11. Mccoy, J.M.; Eckert, J.R.E.F. Sialadenoma papilliferum. *J. Oral Surg.* **1980**, *38*, 691–693. [PubMed]
12. Nasu, M.; Takagi, M.; Ishikawa, G. Sialoadenoma papilliferum. Report of a case. *J. Oral Surg.* **1981**, *39*, 367–369. [PubMed]
13. Wertheimer, F.W.; Bank, K.; Ruskin, W.J. Sialadenoma papilliferum. *Int. J. Oral Surg.* **1983**, *12*, 190–193. [CrossRef]
14. Puts, J.J.; Voorsmit, R.A.; Van Haelst, U.J. Sialocystadenoma papilliferum of the palate. *J. Maxillofac. Surg.* **1984**, *12*, 904. [CrossRef]
15. Rennie, J.S.; MacDonald, D.G.; Critchlow, H.A. Sialadenoma papilliferum. A case report and review of the literature. *Int. J. Oral Surg.* **1984**, *13*, 452–454. [CrossRef]
16. Shirasuna, K.; Watatani, K.; Mlyazakl, T. Ultrastructure of a sialoadenoma papilliferum. *Cancer* **1984**, *53*, 468–474. [CrossRef]
17. Bass, K.D.; Cosentino, B.J. Sialadenoma papilliferum. *J. Oral Maxillofac. Surg.* **1985**, *43*, 302–304. [CrossRef]
18. Regezi, J.A.; Lloyd, R.V.; Zarbo, R.J.; Mcclatchey, K.D. Minor salivary gland tumors. A histologic and immunohisto chemical study. *Cancer* **1985**, *55*, 108–115. [CrossRef]
19. Fantasia, J.E.; Nocco, C.E.; Lally, E.T. Ultrastructureof sialadenoma papilliferum. *Arch. Pathol. Lab. Med.* **1986**, *110*, 523–527.
20. Mitre, B.K. Sialoadenoma papilliferum: Report of case and review of literature. *J. Oral Maxillofac. Surg.* **1986**, *44*, 469–474. [CrossRef]
21. Papanicolaou, S.J.; Triantafyllou, A.G. Sialadenoma papilliferam of the oral cavity: A case report and review of the literature. *J. Oral Med.* **1987**, *42*, 57. [PubMed]

22. Van der Wal, J.E.; Van der Waal, I. The rare sialadenoma papilliferum: Report of a case and review of the literature. *Int. J. Oral Maxillofac. Surg.* **1992**, *21*, 104–106. [CrossRef]
23. Pimentel, M.T.; Lopez Amado, M.; Garcia, S.A. Recurrent sialadenoma papilliferum of the buccal mucosa. *J. Laryngol. Otol.* **1995**, *109*, 787–790. [CrossRef] [PubMed]
24. Maiorano, E.; Favia, G.; Ricco, R. Sialadenoma papilliferum: An immunohistochemical study of five cases. *J. Oral Pathol. Med.* **1996**, *25*, 336–342. [CrossRef]
25. Markopoulos, A.; Kayavis, I.; Papanayotou, P. Sialadenoma papilliferum of the oral cavity: Report of a case and literature review. *J. Oral Maxillofac. Surg.* **1997**, *55*, 1181–1184. [CrossRef]
26. Asahina, I.; Masato, A. Sialadenoma papilliferum of the hard palate: A case report of a case and review of literature. *J. Oral Maxillofac. Surg.* **1997**, *55*, 1000–1003. [CrossRef]
27. Argyres, M.I.; Golitz, L.E. Sialadenoma papilliferum of the palate: Case report and literature review. *J. Cutan. Pathol.* **1999**, *26*, 259–262. [CrossRef]
28. Brannon, R.B.; Sciubba, J.J.; Giulani, M. Ductal papillomas of salivary gland origin: A report of 19 cases and a review of the literature. *Oral Surg. Oral Med. Oral Pathol. Oral Radiol. Endod.* **2001**, *92*, 68–77. [CrossRef]
29. Ubaidat, M.A.; Robinson, R.A.; Belding, P.J.; Merryman, D.J. Sialadenoma papilliferum of the hard palate: Report of 2 cases and immunohistochemical evaluation. *Arch. Pathol. Lab. Med.* **2001**, *125*, 1595–1597. [CrossRef]
30. Shimoda, M.; Kameyama, K.; Morinaga, S.; Tanaka, Y.; Hashiguchu, K.; Shimada, M.; Okara, Y. Malignant transformation of sialadenoma papilliferum of the palate: A case report. *Virchows Arch.* **2004**, *445*, 641–646. [CrossRef]
31. Gomes, A.P.; Sobral, A.P.; Loducca, S.V.; de Araujo, V.C. Sialadenoma papilliferum: Immunohistochemical study. *Int. J. Oral Maxillofac. Surg.* **2004**, *33*, 621–624. [CrossRef] [PubMed]
32. Mahajan, D.; Khurana, N.; Setia, N. Sialadenoma papilliferum in a young patient: A case report and review of the literature. *Oral Surg. Oral Med. Oral Pathol. Oral Radiol. Endod.* **2007**, *103*, 51–54. [CrossRef] [PubMed]
33. Ponniah, I. A rare case of sialadenoma papilliferum with epithelial dysplasia and carcinoma in situ. *Oral Surg. Oral Med. Oral Pathol. Oral Radiol. Endod.* **2007**, *104*, 27–29. [CrossRef] [PubMed]
34. Vicente, O.P.; Marques, N.A.; Aytes, L.B.; Escoda, C.G. Minor salivary gland tumors: A clinicopathological study of 18 cases. *Med. Oral Patol. Oral Cir. Bucal.* **2008**, *13*, 582–588.
35. Liu, W.; Gnepp, D.R.; de Vries, E.; Bibawy, H.; Solomon, M.; Gloster, E.S. Mucoepidermoid carcinoma arising in a background of sialadenoma papilliferum: A case report. *Head Neck Pathol.* **2009**, *3*, 59–62. [CrossRef]
36. Ide, F.; Kikuchi, K.; Kusama, K.; Kanazawa, H. Sialadenoma papilliferum with potentially malignant features. *J. Clin. Pathol.* **2010**, *63*, 362–364. [CrossRef]
37. Kubota, Y.; Kubo, C.; Mori, Y. Sialadenoma Papilliferum of the Hard Palate: A Case Report. *J. Oral Maxillofac. Surg.* **2011**, *70*, 1609–1612. [CrossRef]
38. Anuradha, A.; Ram Prasad, V.V.; Kashyap, B.; Srinivas, V. Sialadenoma papilliferum: Clinical misdiagnosis with a histological decree. *Case Rep. Dent.* **2012**, *2012*, 356271. [CrossRef]
39. Reis de Sá Silva e Costa, F.E.; Vizcaíno Vázquez, J.R. Sialadenoma Papilliferum with inverted pattern in a young patient: A case report. *Am. J. Case Rep.* **2015**, *16*, 663–666. [CrossRef]
40. Santos, J.N.; Barros, A.C.; Gurgel, C.A.; Ramalho, L.M.P. Sialadenoma papilliferum of the tongue mimicking a malignant tumor. *Braz. J. Otorhinolaryngol.* **2013**, *79*, 404. [CrossRef]
41. Fowler, C.B.; Damm, D.D. Sialadenoma Papilliferum: Analysis of Seven New Cases and Review of the Literature. *Head Neck Pathol.* **2018**, *12*, 193–201. [CrossRef] [PubMed]
42. Miyamoto, S.; Ogawa, T.; Chikazu, D. Sialadenoma papilliferum in the buccal mucosa detected on (18)F-fluorodeoxyglucose-positron emission tomography. *Br. J. Oral Maxillofac. Surg.* **2017**, *55*, 727–729. [CrossRef] [PubMed]
43. Sunil, S.; Babu, S.S.; Panicker, S.; Pratap, N. Sialadenoma papilliferum: A rare case report and review of literature. *J. Cancer Res. Ther.* **2017**, *13*, 148–151. [CrossRef] [PubMed]
44. Atarbashi-Moghadam, S.; Lotfi, A.; Moshref, M.; Mokhtari, S. Sialadenoma papilliferum of the hard palate: A rare case report. *Indian J. Pathol. Microbiol.* **2019**, *62*, 163–164. [PubMed]
45. Kronenberg, J.; Horowitz, A.; Leventon, G. Sialoadenoma papilliferum of the parotid gland. *J. Laryngol. Otol.* **1989**, *103*, 1089–1090. [CrossRef]
46. Loehn, B.; Sutton, C.; Jastram-Belcher, J.; Harton, A.; Anderson, D.; Walvekar, R.R. Sialadenoma papilliferum of the parotid gland: Case report and review of literature. *Head Neck* **2013**, *35*, E74–E76. [CrossRef]
47. Grushka, M.; Podoshin, L.; Boss, J.H.; Fradis, M. Sialadenoma papilliferum of the parotid gland. *Laryngoscope* **1984**, *94*, 231–233. [CrossRef]
48. Takasugi, N.; Yoshida, H.; Tani, M.; Ikeda, H.; Kitayoshi, M.; Iseki, T.; Akiyama, H.; Kotaki, S.; Ikeda, C.; Tominaga, K. Sialadenoma papilliferum: Special staining and immunohistochemical staining. *J. Oral Maxillofac. Surg.* **2021**, *33*, 358–361. [CrossRef]
49. Melo, G.M.; Cervantes, O.; Abrahao, M.; Covolan, L.; Ferreira, E.S.; Baptista, H.A. A brief history of salivary gland surgery. *Rev. Colégio Bras. Cir.* **2017**, *44*, 403–412. [CrossRef]
50. Hsieh, M.S.; Bishop, J.A.; Yu Fong Chang, J. Sialadenoma Papilliferum. *Surg. Pathol. Clin.* **2021**, *14*, 43–51. [CrossRef]
51. Vaidya, A.D.; Pantvaidya, G.H.; Metgudmath, R.; Kane, S.V.; D'Cruz, A.K. Minor salivary gland tumors of the oral cavity: A case series with review of literature. *J. Cancer Res. Ther.* **2012**, *8* (Suppl. S1), S111–S115. [PubMed]

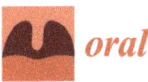

Article

Onset of MRONJ in Breast Cancer Patients after Switching from Low to High Dose of Bone Modifying Agents Due to Bone Metastases Development: A Single Center Retrospective Cohort Study

Rodolfo Mauceri [1,*], Martina Coppini [1] and Giuseppina Campisi [2]

1 Department of Surgical, Oncological and Oral Sciences, University of Palermo, 90127 Palermo, Italy
2 Unit of Oral Medicine and Dentistry for Fragile Patients, Department of Rehabilitation, Fragility and Continuity of Care, University Hospital Palermo, 90127 Palermo, Italy
* Correspondence: rodolfo.mauceri@unipa.it

Abstract: Background: Medication-Related Osteonecrosis of the Jaw (MRONJ) is an adverse drug reaction mainly associated to bone modifying agents (BMAs). Breast cancer (BC) is the most frequent cancer worldwide. Its therapy can cause cancer treatment-induced bone loss (CTIBL), commonly treated with BMAs. The aims of this retrospective study are: to describe characteristics of BC patients under BMAs for CTIBL; to record any switch to high-dose BMAs; to assess MRONJ onset and to identify any factors associated with it. Patients: Authors included patients referred for MRONJ prevention to the Unit of Oral Medicine (University Hospital of Palermo). Results: Fourteen female BC patients under low-dose BMAs for CTIBL were eligible (mean age 66.6 years). Four patients switched to high-dose BMAs for bone metastases. In two of the four, MRONJ developed: one case, in the mandible (risedronate for 48 months then Xgeva® for 60 months); the other case, in the maxilla (Prolia® for 20 months then zoledronate for 16 months). Conclusion: It can be theorized that BC patients under BMAs for CTIBL are likely to have MRONJ risk similar to osteo-metabolic patients. These patients need more careful monitoring of oral health since they may switch, for preventing or treating bone metastases, to heavier BMAs therapy, thus increasing their risk of MRONJ.

Keywords: osteonecrosis of the jaw; MRONJ; cancer treatment-induced bone loss; CTIBL; breast cancer; osteoporosis; bone metastases; bisphosphonates; BPs; denosumab

1. Introduction

Medication-Related Osteonecrosis of the Jaw (MRONJ) can be defined as "adverse drug reaction described as the progressive destruction and death of bone that affects the mandible and maxilla of patients exposed to the treatment with medications known to increase the risk of disease, in the absence of a previous radiation treatment", to be diagnosed and scored by clinics and radiological exams, independently from the presence of exposed necrotic bone or bone probing via sinus/fistula tracts for more than 8 weeks [1,2].

MRONJ is considered a potentially serious complication mainly of bone modifying agents (BMAs) treatment in patients with bone metastases (BM) due to various cancers and with multiple myeloma, as well as osteoporosis [3]. MRONJ may also develop in BMAs-naive patients exposed to a variety of anti-angiogenic agents [4–6].

Breast cancer (BC) is the world's most prevalent cancer. In 2020, there were 2.3 million women diagnosed with BC and 685,000 deaths globally. BC has a prevalence estimated in 2020 (time period 5 years) of 7.8 million women [7,8].

In patients affected by BC, since early menopause is induced by gonadotropin-releasing hormone analogues or chemotherapy and/or aromatase inhibitors reduce estrogen levels, there is the risk of developing Cancer Treatment-Induced Bone Loss (CTIBL), apart from

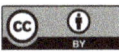

the further risk of developing BM in advanced stages of BC [8]. The drugs of choice for CTIBL prevention are BMAs, such as bisphosphonates (BPs) or denosumab (DNB) [9,10].

In RCTs on BC patients, treated with low doses of BMAs for CTIBL prevention, the onset of MRONJ was observed between 0% and 10.4%, but data are very scarce and debatable [11–14].

This retrospective cohort study aims to: (i) describe the characteristics of BC patients under BMAs for CTIBL prevention in dental follow-up; (ii) record any switching to high dose BMAs therapy; (iii) assess the onset of MRONJ; and (iv) identify the factors associated with MRONJ.

2. Materials and Methods

2.1. Study Design

The following observational cohort study was approved by the Institutional Local Ethics Committee of the University Hospital "P. Giaccone" of Palermo, Palermo, Italy (approval number 1/2022). The study was conducted according to the Principles of the Declaration of Helsinki on experimentation involving human subjects and a written informed consent was obtained from all participants. The study was performed following the STROBE Statement for Observational Cohort Studies. Authors consecutively included all the BC patients scheduled to receive BMAs therapy or already in BMAs therapy for CTIBL and referred to Unit of Oral Medicine of the University Hospital of Palermo from December 2015 to February 2020. For each patient, demographic data, number and type of BMA therapies, onset of bone metastases, diagnosis of systemic, drug-related and local risk factors (e.g., diabetes, corticosteroids, periodontitis) and smoking habits were recorded. All these patients underwent oral examination and dedicated radiological investigation (e.g., orthopantomography—OPT) and, when necessary, computed tomography (CT) or cone beam CT (CBCT).

2.2. Eligibility Criteria

The patients were selected based on the following inclusion criteria:
- patients suffering from BC commencing, taking or who had taken BMAs for CTIBL
- at least 12 months of dental follow-up.

The exclusion criteria were: patients with different cancer or BC and metastases; patients receiving off-label use of BMAs; patients receiving anti-angiogenic drugs alone or in combination with BMAs; patients who underwent radiant therapy head-neck district or were affected by jaws cancer or metastases.

2.3. Outcome Measures

For each patient, the following data were recorded: demographic data, any systemic, drug-related (i.e., type, duration and formulation of BMAs), and local risk factors (e.g., diabetes, corticosteroids, periodontitis), smoking habits, site of each MRONJ lesion, and clinical-radiological stage by SICMF-SIPMO [2,15].

MRONJ has been diagnosed according to the SICMF-SIPMO recommendation, by means of CT or CBCT [2,15].

2.4. Statistical Analysis

The onset of MRONJ was considered as the primary outcome variable and expressed dichotomously. The type of cancer, reason for BMAs treatment, the type of drug, the duration of therapy as well as drug-suspension were expressed as frequencies and percentages. Age was reported as mean and standard deviation.

3. Results

Characteristics of Patients

Fourteen patients with breast cancer (BC) under low dose of BMAs for CTIBL prevention were eligible. Data have been collected and Table 1 illustrates the characteristics of patients at the baseline.

All patients were female and affected by BC, with a mean age of 66.6 (±11.9 years, range 48–84 years). Seven patients (7/14, 50%) had various comorbidities: five hypertension (35.7%), two arthrosis (14.3%), two diabetes mellitus (14.3%). Twelve patients had local risk factors: poor oral hygiene, periodontal disease, endo-periodontal lesion, and dental prosthesis). Only one patient was a smoker (1/14, 7.1%) (Table 1).

In the first dental visit all patients were assuming low dose BMAs, specifically: alendronate 6/14 (42,9%), clodronate 6/14 (42,9%), risedronate 1/14 (7,1%), Prolia® (DNB 60 mg/biannually) 1/14 (7,1%). Among patients assuming clodronate, one patient had a previous history of alendronate intake. The median number of months of low dose BMAs was 57.9 (+47.1 months) (Table 2).

All patients were subjected to primary and secondary prevention measures for MRONJ.

During the follow-up period (median follow-up period 28.1 ± 19.6 months), out of 14 patients, 4 patients switched from low dose BMAs to high dose BMAs due to the development of bone metastasis (4/14, 28.6%). The mean time from the assumption of low dose to high dose BMAs was 35 months (± 15.1 months). Three patients switched from BPs to Xgeva® (DNB 120 mg/month), one patient switched from Prolia® to zoledronate (e.v.). The median number of months of Xgeva® was 28 (±23.6, 4–60); one patient assumed zoledronate (e.v.) for 16 months (Table 2). Among these four patients, two developed MRONJ (2/4, 50%) (2/14, 14.3%) (Figure 1, Tables 3 and 4).

Seven patients (50%) underwent dental extractions for MRONJ primary prevention (four patients assuming low dose BMAs; three assuming high dose BMAs). Overall, 15 extractions were made: 10 (66.6%) were from the maxilla (2 anterior teeth, 8 posterior teeth) and 5 (33.3%) from the mandible (all posterior teeth). A drug suspension protocol for medications at risk was observed in 85.7% of cases (6/7 patients) when dental surgery was considered necessary. None of these patients developed MRONJ in the post-extraction site. During the follow-up period, one patient changed low dose BMA from alendronate to Prolia®. The two patients that developed MRONJ underwent surgical therapy of MRONJ, both patients healed.

Table 1. Characteristics of enrolled breast cancer patients.

Patient	Age	Systemic Disease	Local Risk Factors	ONJ-Related Drugs	Duration (Months)	Cumulative Doses (mg)	Dental Extractions	N. Teeth Extracted	MRONJ Onset during Follow-Up	Time-Lapse between 1st° Visit and Last Check-Up (Months)
#1	53	Autoimmune thyroiditis	Poor oral hygiene, dental prosthesis	alendronate clodronate	48 12	13,440 2400	No	n.a.	No	12
#2	79	Arthrosis, diabetes	Poor oral hygiene	clodronate	120	24,000	No	n.a.	No	14
#3	73	Hypertension, arthrosis, diabetes, hepatitis C	Poor oral hygiene	clodronate	82	16,400	No	n.a.	No	19
#4	83	n.a.	Poor oral hygiene	clodronate	132	26,400	No	n.a.	No	12
#5	75	n.a.	Dental prosthesis, periodontal disease, poor oral hygiene, endo-periodontal lesion	risedronate Xgeva®	48 60	7200 7200	Yes	2	Yes	84
#6	57	Hypertension, osteomalacia	endo-periodontal lesion	alendronate	12	3360	Yes	2	No	42
#7	70	Hypertension	Dental prosthesis, periodontal disease, poor oral hygiene	alendronate	156	43,680	Yes	1	No	36
#8	48	Thalassaemia carrier	n.a.	alendronate	33	9240	Yes	2	No	40
#9	67	N.a.	n.a.	clodronate	12	2400	No	n.a.	No	12
#10	71	Hepatitis C	Periodontal disease, poor oral hygiene	alendronate Xgeva®	48 4	13,440 480	Yes	4	No	30
#11	51	Hypertension	Dental prosthesis	alendronate Prolia®	20 12	5600 120	Yes	3	No	23
#12	84	Hypertension	Poor oral hygiene	clodronate Xgeva®	24 20	4800 2400	No	n.a.	No	12
#13	56	N.a.	Periodontal disease, poor oral hygiene	Prolia® zoledronate	20 16	180 64	Yes	3	Yes	21
#14	66	N.a.	Dental prosthesis, periodontal disease, poor oral hygiene	alendronate	44	3360	No	n.a.	No	36

Table 2. Details of BMA therapy.

	Number of Patients	Median and Standard Deviation	%
Low dose BMA for CTIBL	14		
alendronate	6	-	42.9%
clodronate	6	-	42.9%
risedronate	1	-	7.1%
Prolia®	1	-	7.1%
Duration of low dose BMAs therapy (mths)		57.9 (±47.1)	-
High dose BMA for BM	4		
zoledronate	1	-	25%
Xgeva®	3	-	75%
Duration of DNB therapy (mths)	3	28 (±23.6)	-
Duration of ZOL therapy (mths)	1	16	-

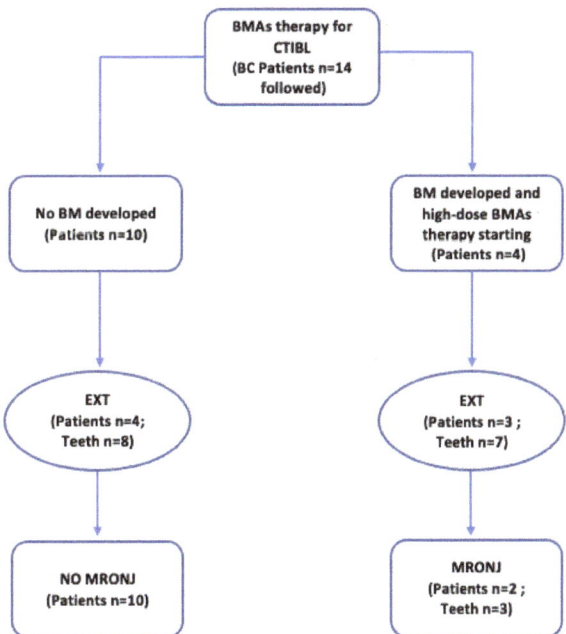

Figure 1. Flow chart of MRONJ occurrence. A relationship between BMAs therapy and MRONJ development after teeth extractions was diagnosed in 14 patients with breast cancer. Four patients developed BM and switched from low dose BMAs to high dose BMAs. Three of these patients underwent dental extractions and two developed MRONJ. Abbreviations: BMAs: Bone Modifying Agents; CTIBL: Cancer Treatment-induced Bone Loss; BM: bone metastases; EXT: extraction.

Table 3. Details of patients affected by breast cancer that switched BMAs therapy due to bone metastases development.

Patient	Age	Sex	MTS	MRONJ after the Pharmacological Switch	ONJ-Related Drgs	Duration (Months)	Cumulative Dosi (mg)	ONJ Localization	ONJ Stage According to SIPMO-SICMF[3]	ONJ Stage According to AAOMS[16]	Clinical Features
#1	75	F	Yes	Yes	risedronate Xgeva®	48 60	7200 7200	Anterior lower jaw	I		Intraoral Fistula, Tooth mobility
#2	56	F	Yes	Yes	Prolia® zoledronate	20 16	180 64	Posterior upper jaw	I		Tooth mobility
#3	71	F	Yes	No	alendronate Xgeva®	48 4	13,440 480	n.a.	n.a.	n.a.	n.a.
#4	84	F	Yes	No	clodronate Xgeva®	24 20	4800 2400	n.a.	n.a.	n.a.	n.a.

Table 4. Differences between BC patients' subgroups.

Characteristics		Patients under Only Low Dose BMAs (No Case of MRONJ)	Patients under Low + High Dose BMAs (No Case of MRONJ)	Patients under Low + High Dose BMAs (Onset of MRONJ)
N patients		10	2	2
Age	Range	48–83	71–84	56–75
	Median	65.5	77.5	65.5
	Standard deviation	11.7	9.2	13.4
Smoking habit		1	0	0
Systemic disease	Hypertension	4	1	0
	Diabetes	2	0	0
	Arthrosis	2	0	0

Table 4. *Cont.*

Characteristics		Patients under Only Low Dose BMAs (No Case of MRONJ)	Patients under Low + High Dose BMAs (No Case of MRONJ)	Patients under Low + High Dose BMAs (Onset of MRONJ)
Local risk factors	Poor oral hygiene	7	2	2
	Dental prosthesis	4	0	1
	Periodontal disease	2	2	1
	Endo-periodontal lesion	1	0	1
Bone MTS		0	2	2
Low dose MRONJ- related drugs durations (months)		67.1 (±52.9)	36 (±17) case #1: 48 mths case#2: 24 mths	34 (±19.8) case #1: 48 mths case#2: 20 mths
Low dose MRONJ- related drugs cumulative dose (mg)		14,788 (±13,286.3)	9120 (±6109.4) case #1: 13,440 mg case #2: 4800 mg	3690 (±4963.9) case #1: 7200 mg case #2: 180 mg
High dose MRONJ- related drugs durations (months)		n.a.	12 (±11.3) Case #1: 4 mths Case#2: 20 mths	38 (±31.1) Case #1: 60 mths Case#2: 16 mths
High dose MRONJ- related drugs cumulative dose (mg)		n.a.	1440 (±1357.6) Case #1: 480 mg Case #2: 2400 mg	3632 (±5045.9) Case #1: 7200 mg Case #2: 64 mg
Dental surgery	N patients	4 (40%)	1 (50%)	2 (100%)
	N extracted teeth	8	4	3
Jaw	Upper	5	3	2
	Lower	3	1	1
Follow-up (months)		24.6 (±12.6)	21 (±12.7)	52.5 (±44.5)

Below detailed cases of MRONJ are presented:

Case 1 (#5 in Table 1 and #1 in Table 3)

In December 2015, A 75-year-old non-smoker woman was referred for primary prevention of MRONJ. In 2011, the patient had been diagnosed with a BC; in September 2015, she developed bone metastases (BM).

From 2011 to 2015 she had been treated with risedronate (48 months, monthly dosing of 75 mg risedronate on 2 consecutive days). After the development of BM and the dental examination, she was switched to Xgeva®. After 60 months of high dose BMA, she developed non-exposed MRONJ in the mandible (Figure 2a). The intra-oral examination revealed a presence of two intraoral fistulas on the 5th sextant, associated with a rapid onset of teeth mobility (3.1, 3.2, 4.2). The CBCT showed cortical erosion, osteosclerotic pattern, periodontal space widening and bone sequestrum formation (Figure 2b–e), confirming to be MRONJ stage I (according to SICMF-SIPMO) [2,3,15]. Moreover, according to the AAOMS staging system, this was Stage I [16]. MRONJ was surgically treated, and there were no signs of recurrencies in the follow-up period.

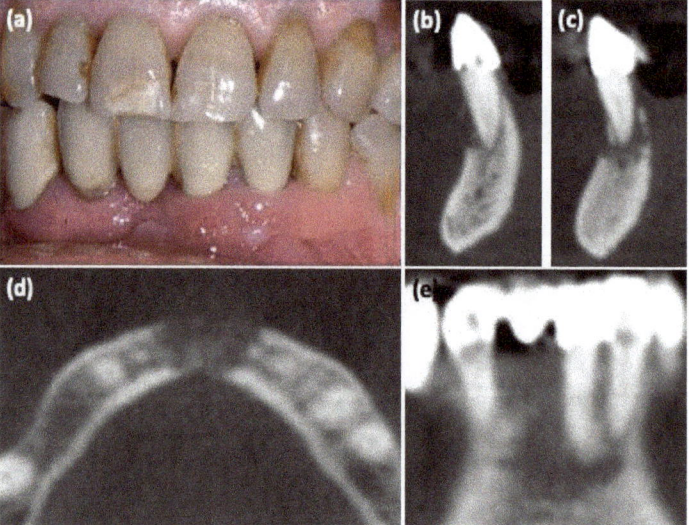

Figure 2. MRONJ stage I, lower jaw: (**a**) clinical view; (**b–e**) computed tomography scan sections.

Case 2 (#13 in Table 1 and #2 in Table 3)

In December 2015, a 56-year-old non-smoker woman was referred for primary prevention of MRONJ. In 2004 BC had been diagnosed; in January 2017 she developed BM.

She was treated from 2015 to 2017 with Prolia® (20 months, DNB 60 mg/biannual). After the development of BM, she was switched to zoledronate (e.v.). After 16 months of high dose BMA she developed non-exposed MRONJ in the mandible (Figure 3a). The intra-oral examination highlighted a presence of the rapid onset of tooth mobility (maxillary right third molar) associated with purulent discharge and pain. CBCT showed a slight osteosclerotic pattern, thickening of the alveolar ridge and sinusitis (Figure 3b,d), confirming to be MRONJ stage I (according to SICMF-SIPMO) [2,3,15]. According to AAOMS, this was Stage II [16]. MRONJ was surgically treated, and an alveolar bone specimen was collected from the interradicular septum during the surgical procedures. MRONJ was histologically confirmed (Figure 3e). There were no signs of recurrencies in the follow-up period.

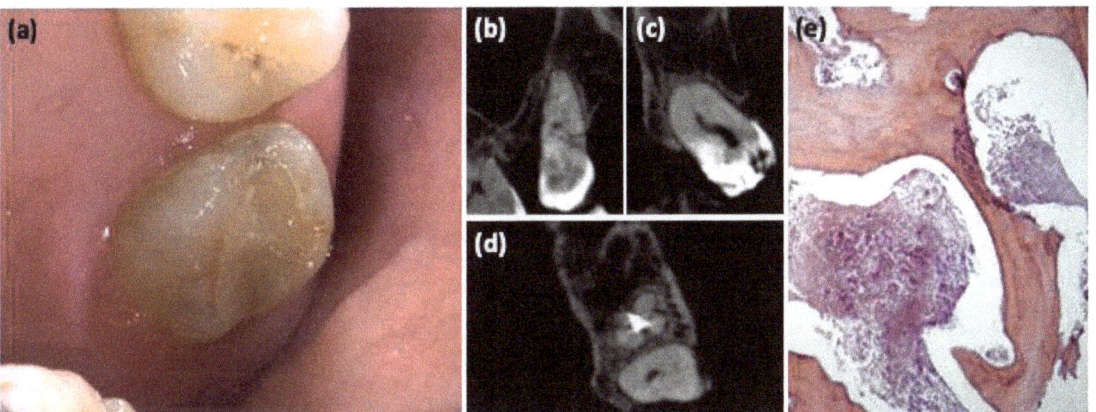

Figure 3. MRONJ stage I, upper jaw: (**a**) clinical view; (**b–d**) computed tomography scan sections; (**e**) magnification of histological findings.

4. Discussion

MRONJ is a rare drug adverse reaction that can greatly affect the quality of the life of patients if not promptly diagnosed and treated [2,17,18].

Based on the literature, it is possible to distinguish, at the least, three main common MRONJ patient populations [2,15]:

(1) *cancer patients with BM or myeloma patients*; generally receiving high dose BMAs often associated with other agents (chemotherapy, endocrine therapy, immunotherapy, antiangiogenics and other biological agents) (high MRONJ risk) [19];

(2) *breast cancer (BC) or prostate cancer patients suffering from osteoporosis without bone metastases receiving bisphosphonates or denosumab to limit the risk of non-metastatic bone fractures (due to CTIBL)*; this population (assuming the same dosage of BMAs) is considered assumable to those with osteoporosis for what concern their MRONJ risk [20];

(3) *patients suffering from osteoporosis and other non-malignant diseases*; receiving BMAs with different regimens (low MRONJ risk) [21];

As previously stated, the first group has been associated to a higher estimation of MRONJ, that was reported between 1% and more than 20% [22,23].

In the second group, composed by breast or prostate cancer patients, without bone metastases and treated with BMAs for the prevention of CTIBL, the incidence of MRONJ was observed between 0% and 10.4% [11–14]. However, data regarding this group of patients are very scarce. Indeed, this group of patients is still poorly known by many clinicians, especially by dentists; this limited knowledge may lead to the possibility of overestimating the risk of MRONJ onset of these patients, if included in cohorts of cancer patients with BM.

The third group is composed by patients suffering from osteoporosis and other non-malignant diseases receiving low dose BMAs; in this group the MRONJ risk is described between 0.01% and 5.2% [24].

Breast cancer is the most frequent tumor in women worldwide, regardless of age, with a peak of incidence in postmenopausal age. CTIBL has been found to be the most common long-term adverse event experienced by breast cancer patients. BPs and DNB are the two classes of BMAs used in clinical practice with similar efficacy in preventing CTIBL and similar issues to be solved, such as the best time of starting BMAs therapy and its duration [20].

All patients at risk of MRONJ should be subjected to primary preventive measures (even after commencing BMAs), with the aim to maintain and/or reestablish as soon as possible an acceptable level of oral health. The preventive measures should be done before the administration of ONJ-related medications in cancer patients with BM or multiple myeloma or within the first six months in osteo-metabolic patients. Furthermore, the patients taking BMAs should undergo periodic dental visits for early diagnosis of MRONJ (every four months for cancer patients with BM or multiple myeloma while every six months for osteo-metabolic patients) [2,25].

This study highlights, based on epidemiological data, that breast cancer or prostate cancer patients without BM and treated with low dose BMAs for CTIBL prevention should be considered similar to patients suffering from osteoporosis receiving low dose BMAs (at the same dosage for CTIBL prevention), hence at low risk of MRONJ onset. It is possible to apply them a binary gradient of MRONJ risk, supposed for osteo-metabolic ones [2,25]:

- from the beginning of BMAs administration to within 3 years from the commencing of the treatment, a patient who does not report other MRONJ risk factors (e.g., systemic and/or local) will be classified and considered at low risk of MRONJ.
- if the patient has been in treatment for a period of time longer than 3 years or shorter than 3 years and simultaneously affected by systemic or local risk factors, this patient will bear an incremental and indefinable risk of developing MRONJ, which is linked to one or more additional, reported systemic or local risk factors.

In any case, all non-invasive dental treatments (e.g., restorative dentistry, non-surgical periodontics), as well as surgical procedures which are necessary to eliminate infective outbreaks of MRONJ, are not only considered as *indicated* but also of the utmost importance in reducing the spreading of infectious processes for primary prevention purposes [2,25–27].

If the patient shows a good oral health or after the resolution of inflammatory or infectious process, it is beneficial to plan a six-month follow-up examination in order to maintain the primary prevention program for patients suffering from breast/prostate cancer, treated with low dose BMAs for CTIBL prevention, from osteoporosis or other non-malignant diseases [2,25,28].

It is worthy of note that, if a given cancer patient develops BM before the assumption of high dose BMAs, the oral condition should be re-evaluated by dental examination and when necessary also thanks to a new radiological dental exam. Additionally, cancer patients with BM or multiple myeloma should undergo periodic dental visits every four months.

Among the 14 BC patients included in this study, with a median follow-up period 28.1 ($\pm$19.6) months, only 4 patients developed BM and then they were treated with high dose BMAs. Among the four BC patients with BM, only two developed MRONJ.

One patient, after 48 months of risedronate assumption, had been treated with Xgeva®; 60 months after the switch she developed a non-exposed Stage I MRONJ in the lower jaw. The second patient, after 20 months of Prolia®, had been treated with zoledronate; 17 months after the switch she developed a non-exposed Stage I MRONJ in the upper jaw. Comparing the data of these two patients affected by BM and MRONJ to those with BM without MRONJ, it must be highlighted that the patients with MRONJ took less low-dose BMAs but longer high-dose BMAs (Table 4).

Noteworthy is the fact that both patients developed a non-exposed stage I MRONJ in association with the onset of tooth mobility. This very light and healable condition is probably derived from adequate and continuative primary and secondary prevention measures. The application of periodic follow-up has made it possible to diagnose the disease at the earliest stage, to carry out effective surgical therapies with the following resolution of the disease.

5. Conclusions

The existence at the least of another category of BC patients taking BMAs, for reasons other than contrasting bone metastases, raises the recent need to properly inform principally dentists and to correctly record pharmaceutical data of cancer patients. The aim is to avoid any overestimation of the risk of MRONJ, or worse, an underestimation of the risk in those patients treated with BMAs for bone metastases.

The general aim, in the protection of BC patients' health, is to plan a primary prevention of MRONJ before and while taking BMAs (both low and high doses), as well as secondary prevention (early diagnosis) with the most adequate and effective dental protocols, as being more stringent (e.g., without implants procedures) when the transition to high-dose BMAs is planned and carried out.

The authors suggest that BC patients need more careful and punctual monitoring of oral health since they, due to their frank cancer history, may have to switch, for containing bone metastases, to high dose BMAs therapy, thus increasing their risk of MRONJ.

Author Contributions: Conceptualization, G.C.; methodology, G.C.; validation, G.C.; formal analysis, M.C.; investigation, R.M and G.C.; data curation, M.C. and G.C.; writing—original draft preparation, R.M.; writing—review and editing, G.C.; visualization, R.M. and M.C.; project administration, G.C. All authors have read and agreed to the published version of the manuscript.

Funding: This research received no external funding. R.M. is supported by Ministero dell'Istruzione, dell'Università e della Ricerca (MIUR)—PON-AIM Line 1 (Id. AIM1892002).

Institutional Review Board Statement: The study was conducted in accordance with the Declaration of Helsinki, and approved by the Institutional Local Ethics Committee of the University Hospital "P. Giaccone " of Palermo, Palermo, Italy (approval number 1/2022).

Informed Consent Statement: Informed consent was obtained from all subjects involved in the study.

Data Availability Statement: Not applicable.

Acknowledgments: The authors also thank V. Rodolico (Unipa) for his role in the histological investigation.

Conflicts of Interest: The authors declare no conflict of interest. G.C. declares to have been a scientific expert for Amgen Italia in 2021.

References

1. Bedogni, A.; Campisi, G.; Fusco, V. *Medication Related Osteonecrosis of the Jaw (MRONJ)*; Qeios: London, UK, 2018.
2. Campisi, G.; Mauceri, R.; Bertoldo, F.; Bettini, G.; Biasotto, M.; Colella, G.; Consolo, U.; Di Fede, O.; Favia, G.; Fusco, V.; et al. Medication-related osteonecrosis of jaws (MRONJ) prevention and diagnosis: Italian consensus update 2020. *Int. J. Environ. Res. Public Health* **2020**, *17*, 5998. [CrossRef]
3. Campisi, G.; Fedele, S.; Fusco, V.; Pizzo, G.; Di Fede, O.; Bedogni, A. Epidemiology, clinical manifestations, risk reduction and treatment strategies of jaw osteonecrosis in cancer patients exposed to antiresorptive agents. *Futur. Oncol.* **2014**, *10*, 257–275. [CrossRef] [PubMed]
4. Nicolatou-Galitis, O.; Kouri, M.; Papadopoulou, E.; Vardas, E.; Galiti, D.; Epstein, J.B.; Elad, S.; Campisi, G.; Tsoukalas, N.; Bektas-Kayhan, K.; et al. Osteonecrosis of the jaw related to non-antiresorptive medications: A systematic review. *Support Care Cancer* **2019**, *27*, 383–394. [CrossRef] [PubMed]
5. Schiodt, M.; Otto, S.; Fedele, S.; Bedogni, A.; Nicolatou-Galitis, O.; Guggenberger, R.; Herlofson, B.B.; Ristow, O.; Kofod, T.; Nicolatou-Galitis, O.; et al. Workshop of European task force on medication-related osteonecrosis of the jaw—Current challenges. *Oral Dis.* **2019**, *25*, 1815–1821. [CrossRef]
6. Pimolbutr, K.; Porter, S.; Fedele, S. Osteonecrosis of the Jaw Associated with Antiangiogenics in Antiresorptive-Naïve Patient: A Comprehensive Review of the Literature. *BioMed Res. Int.* **2018**, *2018*, 8071579. [CrossRef] [PubMed]
7. WHO Breast Cancer. Available online: https://www.who.int/news-room/fact-sheets/detail/breast-cancer (accessed on 28 June 2022).
8. Hirbe, A.; Morgan, E.A.; Uluçkan, Ö.; Weilbaecher, K. Powles Skeletal complications of breast cancer therapies. *Clin. Cancer Res.* **2006**, *12 (20 Pt 2)*, 6309s–6314s. [CrossRef] [PubMed]
9. Hadji, P.; Body, J.J.; Aapro, M.S.; Brufsky, A.; Coleman, R.E.; Guise, T.; Lipton, A.; Tubiana-Hulin, M. Practical guidance for the management of aromatase inhibitor-associated bone loss. *Ann. Oncol.* **2008**, *19*, 1407–1416. [CrossRef] [PubMed]
10. De Sire, A.; Lippi, L.; Venetis, K.; Morganti, S.; Sajjadi, E.; Curci, C.; Ammendolia, A.; Criscitiello, C.; Fusco, N.; Invernizzi, M. Efficacy of Antiresorptive Drugs on Bone Mineral Density in Post-Menopausal Women with Early Breast Cancer Receiving Adjuvant Aromatase Inhibitors: A Systematic Review of Randomized Controlled Trials. *Front. Oncol.* **2022**, *11*, 829875. [CrossRef]
11. Brufsky, A.M.; Harker, W.G.; Beck, J.T.; Bosserman, L.; Vogel, C.; Seidler, C.; Jin, L.; Warsi, G.; Argonza-Aviles, E.; Hohneker, J.; et al. Final 5-year results of Z-FAST trial: Adjuvant zoledronic acid maintains bone mass in postmenopausal breast cancer patients receiving letrozole. *Cancer* **2012**, *118*, 1192–1201. [CrossRef]
12. Coleman, R.; De Boer, R.; Eidtmann, H.; Llombart, A.; Davidson, N.; Neven, P.; Von Minckwitz, G.; Sleeboom, H.P.; Forbes, J.; Barrios, C.; et al. Zoledronic acid (zoledronate) for postmenopausal women with early breast cancer receiving adjuvant letrozole (ZO-FAST study): Final 60-month results. *Ann. Oncol.* **2013**, *24*, 398–405. [CrossRef] [PubMed]

13. Rugani, P.; Luschin, G.; Jakse, N.; Kirnbauer, B.; Lang, U.; Acham, S. Prevalence of bisphosphonate-associated osteonecrosis of the jaw after intravenous zoledronate infusions in patients with early breast cancer. *Clin. Oral Investig.* **2014**, *18*, 401–407. [CrossRef]
14. Gnant, M.; Pfeiler, G.; Steger, G.G.; Egle, D.; Greil, R.; Fitzal, F.; Wette, V.; Balic, M.; Haslbauer, F.; Melbinger-Zeinitzer, E.; et al. Adjuvant denosumab in postmenopausal patients with hormone receptor-positive breast cancer (ABCSG-18): Disease-free survival results from a randomised, double-blind, placebo-controlled, phase 3 trial. *Lancet Oncol.* **2019**, *20*, 339–351. [CrossRef]
15. Campisi, G.; Bedogni, A.; Fusco, V. *Raccomandazioni Clinico-Terapeutiche Sull'osteonecrosi Delle Ossa Mascellari (ONJ) Farmaco-Relata E Sua Prevenzione*; Srl, N.D.F., Ed.; Palermo University Press: Palermo, Italy, 2020; ISBN 978-88-5509-148-0.
16. Ruggiero, S.L.; Dodson, T.B.; Fantasia, J.; Goodday, R.; Aghaloo, T.; Mehrotra, B.; O'Ryan, F. American Association of Oral and Maxillofacial Surgeons position paper on medication-related osteonecrosis of the jaw—2014 update. *J. Oral Maxillofac. Surg.* **2014**, *72*, 1938–1956. [CrossRef]
17. Oteri, G.; De Ponte, F.S.; Runci, M.; Peditto, M.; Marcianò, A.; Cicciù, M. Oral-Health-Related Quality of Life After Surgical Treatment of Osteonecrosis of the Jaws. *J. Craniofac. Surg.* **2017**, *29*, 403–408. [CrossRef]
18. El-Rabbany, M.; Lam, D.K.; Shah, P.S.; Azarpazhooh, A. Surgical Management of Medication-Related Osteonecrosis of the Jaw Is Associated with Improved Disease Resolution: A Retrospective Cohort Study. *J. Oral Maxillofac. Surg.* **2019**, *77*, 1816–1822. [CrossRef] [PubMed]
19. Srivastava, A.; Nogueras Gonzalez, G.M.; Geng, Y.; Won, A.M.; Cabanillas, M.E.; Naing, A.; Myers, J.N.; Li, Y.; Chambers, M.S. Prevalence of medication related osteonecrosis of the jaw in patients treated with sequential antiresorptive drugs: Systematic review and meta-analysis. *Support Care Cancer* **2021**, *29*, 2305–2317. [CrossRef]
20. Diana, A.; Carlino, F.; Giunta, E.F.; Franzese, E.; Guerrera, L.P.; Di Lauro, V.; Ciardiello, F.; Daniele, B.; Orditura, M. Cancer Treatment–Induced Bone Loss (CTIBL): State of the Art and Proper Management in Breast Cancer Patients on Endocrine Therapy. *Curr. Treat. Options Oncol.* **2021**, *22*, 45. [CrossRef]
21. Kawahara, M.; Kuroshima, S.; Sawase, T. Clinical considerations for medication-related osteonecrosis of the jaw: A comprehensive literature review. *Int. J. Implant Dent.* **2021**, *7*, 47. [CrossRef]
22. Hortobagyi, G.N.; Van Poznak, C.; Harker, W.G.; Gradishar, W.J.; Chew, H.; Dakhil, S.R.; Haley, B.B.; Sauter, N.; Mohanlal, R.; Zheng, M.; et al. Continued treatment effect of zoledronic acid dosing every 12 vs. 4 weeks in women with breast cancer metastatic to bone: The OPTIMIZE-2 randomized clinical trial. *JAMA Oncol.* **2017**, *3*, 906–912. [CrossRef]
23. Hata, H.; Imamachi, K.; Ueda, M.; Matsuzaka, M.; Hiraga, H.; Osanai, T.; Harabayashi, T.; Fujimoto, K.; Oizumi, S.; Takahashi, M.; et al. Prognosis by cancer type and incidence of zoledronic acid–related osteonecrosis of the jaw: A single-center retrospective study. *Support. Care Cancer* **2022**, *30*, 4505–4514. [CrossRef] [PubMed]
24. Mavrokokki, T.; Cheng, A.; Stein, B.; Goss, A. Nature and frequency of bisphosphonate-associated osteonecrosis of the jaws in Australia. *J. Oral Maxillofac. Surg.* **2007**, *65*, 415–423. [CrossRef] [PubMed]
25. Di Fede, O.; Panzarella, V.; Mauceri, R.; Fusco, V.; Bedogni, A.; Lo Muzio, L.; Sipmo Onj Board; Campisi, G. The dental management of patients at risk of medication-related osteonecrosis of the jaw: New paradigm of primary prevention. *Biomed. Res. Int.* **2018**, *2018*, 2684924. [CrossRef] [PubMed]
26. Nicolatou-Galitis, O.; Razis, E.; Galiti, D.; Galitis, E.; Labropoulos, S.; Tsimpidakis, A.; Sgouros, J.; Karampeazis, A.; Migliorati, C. Periodontal disease preceding osteonecrosis of the jaw (ONJ) in cancer patients receiving antiresorptives alone or combined with targeted therapies: Report of 5 cases and literature review. *Oral Surg. Oral Med. Oral Pathol. Oral Radiol.* **2015**, *120*, 699–706. [CrossRef]
27. Soutome, S.; Otsuru, M.; Hayashida, S.; Murata, M.; Yanamoto, S.; Sawada, S.; Kojima, Y.; Funahara, M.; Iwai, H.; Umeda, M.; et al. Relationship between tooth extraction and development of medication-related osteonecrosis of the jaw in cancer patients. *Sci. Rep.* **2021**, *11*, 17226. [CrossRef]
28. Mauceri, R.; Coniglio, R.; Abbinante, A.; Carcieri, P.; Tomassi, D.; Panzarella, V.; Di Fede, O.; Bertoldo, F.; Fusco, V.; Bedogni, A.; et al. The preventive care of medication-related osteonecrosis of the jaw (MRONJ): A position paper by Italian experts for dental hygienists. *Support. Care Cancer* **2022**, *30*, 6429–6440. [CrossRef]

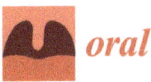 *oral*

Review

Phenotypes, Genotypes, and Treatment Options of Primary Failure of Eruption: A Narrative Review

Luca Testarelli *, Francesca Sestito, Adriana De Stefano, Chiara Seracchiani, Roberto Vernucci and Gabriella Galluccio

Department of Oral and Maxillo Facial Sciences, Sapienza University of Rome, 00161 Rome, Italy
* Correspondence: luca.testarelli@uniroma1.it; Tel.: +39-06-4997-8140

Abstract: Tooth eruption is a complex process, during which a series of factors can cause a failure of it. Among this, primary failure of eruption (PFE) is a non-syndromic condition that leads to an incomplete tooth eruption despite the presence of a clear eruption pathway. The aim of this narrative review is to provide an overall view about clinical considerations, genetics-related aspects, and possible treatments of PFE based on the latest findings. A literature search using the PubMed/Medline and Scopus database was performed. The search terms used were "PFE", "orthodontics", "primary failure of eruption", and "treatment", and all the articles, according to the inclusion criteria, from 2008 until June 2022 were screened. Among them, 12 articles were considered useful to highlight some of the main genotypical and phenotypical aspects and several treatment options. Indeed, if there is a suspicion of primary failure of eruption, a *PTH1R* screening should be performed, because a mutation in this gene is responsible for an altered balance between the resorptive and the appositional processes during the eruption. This is important to know before starting an orthodontic treatment because it could lead to ankylosis of the affected tooth, exposing patients to iatrogenic damage. Treatment options depend on the growth phase of the patient and on the clinical situation.

Keywords: PFE; tooth eruption; failure of eruption; eruption disorder

1. Introduction

Tooth eruption is the movement of the tooth towards its functional position in the oral cavity, entering into contact with the opposing tooth of the upper or lower arch from its developmental site within the alveolar process [1]. Three factors contribute to this complex process: bone resorption, gingival resorption, and root elongation at the apex of the follicle [2].

This is a complex process in which the tooth follicle interacts with osteoclasts and osteoblasts [3,4]. The mononuclear cells that inflow into the coronal part of the tooth follicle are responsible for bone resorption [5]. Tooth eruption is known as a localized and genetically programmed process governed by time.

Both systemic and local factors can cause the failure of tooth eruption. When a systemic cause is involved, often the patient is affected by a systemic syndrome. In particular, the genetic disorders associated with tooth eruption failure are cleidocranial dysplasia, osteopetrosis, Rutherford syndrome, ectodermal dysplasia, and Down syndrome [6]. When the patient has one of these complex systemic diseases, many teeth are usually affected. Instead, when the responsible for the failure of eruption is a local factor, usually only single teeth are affected, mainly the upper canine [7] and the lower wisdom teeth [8]. The local factors that hinder the eruption can be the lack of space, tooth germ deformity, abnormal tooth germ position [9], or a physical barrier in the eruption pathway, such as an odontoma, supernumerary teeth, or cysts [6]. This condition is known as mechanical failure of eruption (MFE). In this case, there is a mechanical obstruction on the eruption pathway, whose removal can cause the resolution of the missing eruption [10].

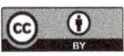

Among the mechanisms of tooth eruption failure, it is important to cite the primary and the secondary retention. In the first case, a dental element, before the emergence in the oral cavity, ceases to erupt in absence of a mechanical obstruction. The secondary retention involves the unexplained cessation of further eruption after a tooth has penetrated the oral mucosa [8,11].

Primary failure of eruption (PFE) [12] is a condition in which non-ankylosed teeth fail to erupt, despite the presence of a clear eruption pathway. Alterations in the balance between the resorptive and the appositional processes during the eruption are the putative factors underlying the development of primary failure of eruption [13]. This condition is generally linked to the mutation of the parathyroid hormone 1 receptor gene (*PTH1R*) [13]. The reviewers decided to focus on the studies conducted from 2008 onwards because in this year articles about the connection between *PTH1R* mutation and PFE were published [14].

Despite several articles having been published in recent years, no review has been recently published that summarizes and organizes the most recent findings about the topic. Starting from the last reviews about PFE, this article has the task of summarizing the latest information based on the most recent research about the genetic bases of primary failure of eruption. Indeed, since the article of Hanisch et al. in 2018, several findings have been introduced, especially regarding the genotypical aspects by Grippaudo et al. in 2018 and 2021. These findings have also changed the clinical approach to PFE. According to this, the aim of the current review is to provide an updated overall view of PFE, from the epidemiology to the treatment going through clinical and genetical aspects.

Furthermore, the research underlines a lack of information about treatment options: further studies are needed to assess which is the best way to treat PFE patients.

2. Materials and Methods

A literature search of the PubMed/Medline and Scopus database, including all English language papers published after 2008 until June 2022, was performed. For the research, the terms used were as follows: "PFE", "Orthodontics", "Treatment", and "Primary failure of eruption". The keywords were combined in several ways: "PFE" AND "Treatment", "PFE" AND "Orthodontics", "Primary failure of eruption" AND "Orthodontics", etc.

The article types selected were systematic reviews, clinical research, clinical randomized studies, and observational studies. Case reports and case series were excluded by this study.

Two calibrated reviewers (FS and CS) independently conducted the search from April to June 2022 and identified 41 articles. After removing the duplicates, just 20 articles remained to be screened. According to the inclusion criteria, the authors examined the articles and removed every study with lower quality of evidence, such as case reports and case studies.

For the eligibility of inclusion, only 12 articles were selected and analyzed.

3. Results

The subjects of the 12 different articles included and discussed in the current narrative review have been summarized in Table 1. Ten out twelve articles discussed the genotypical aspects of PFE, eight out of twelve discussed phenotypes, five out of twelve discussed the epidemiological aspects, and only three out of twelve (25%) discussed the treatment options. To be more precise, Stellzig-Eisenhauer et al. (2013) [6], Milani et al. (2014) [15], Hanisch et al. (2018) [16], Tokavanich et al. (2020) [17], and Grippaudo et al. (2021) [10] provide a general view of the epidemiology of PFE. Each of the selected articles considers the genotypical aspects and the correlation between *PTH1R* mutation and primary failure of eruption except for the articles by Stellzig-Eisenhauer et al. (2013) [6] and Rizzo et al. (2020) [18]. Regarding the phenotypical aspects, Stellzig-Eisenhauer et al. (2013) [6], Izumida et al. (2020) [19], Tokavanich et al. (2020) [17], and Rizzo et al. (2020) [18] did not expose new findings about the clinical and phenotypical aspects of this complex pathology. Unfortunately, in the above mentioned studies, treatment options are not as well treated as every other aspect: only Milani et al. (2014) [15], Hanisch et al. (2018) [16], and Rizzo et al. (2020) [18] debate this topic.

4. Discussion

As stated by Baccetti in 2000, primary failure of eruption is a rare disease with a prevalence of 0.06% [20]. Several published studies of different authors in several countries confirmed the abovementioned percentage [6,16]. On the other hand, the data about gender distribution are not unanimous: several studies confirm the findings of Baccetti's article, in which he reported a prevalence ratio of 1:2.25 (male:female) for PFE [20]. In contrast, Stellzig-Eisenhauer et al. [6], in the sample analyzed, found a 1:1.1 distribution between females and males. Maybe this difference could be related to the small size analyzed in the previously mentioned study. Considering the important contrast observed between these studies, further research is required to accurately assess the gender prevalence of PFE. In all the reported cases of the studies selected, only molars or molars and premolars were involved [21]. This observation could lead to the conclusion that only molars and premolars can be affected by PFE. Hanisch et al. [16] observed a prevalence of 64.1% for the bilateral distribution and a prevalence of 35.9% for the unilateral distribution. A prevalence for the unilateral distribution can be observed also in the impacted second molars [22]. On the other hand, in the article by Pilz et al. (2014), the ratio of bilateral versus unilateral PFE was 20:3. Pilz et al. stated that PFE is usually asymmetric, which means there is a bilaterally unbalanced eruption of the teeth. In other words, the presentation is more severe on one of the two sides [23]. The permanent dentition is more affected than the deciduous dentition [16]. This epidemiological difference can probably be explained by the small sample size of the abovementioned study. For this reason, further studies are needed to better examine the exact gender prevalence and the lateral or bilateral distribution.

There are different types of PFE [17]. In type 1, patients show a similar loss of eruption potential of all affected teeth, which leads to a progressively open bite extending from anterior to posterior. In the second type, the tooth distal to the furthest mesial involved tooth exhibits larger, but still inadequate, eruption potential. In Type 3, both forms appear in the various quadrants.

Proffit and Vig in 1981 [12] identified the following characteristics typical of PFE: involved teeth may initially erupt and then cease to erupt further or may fail to erupt entirely. Therefore, the non-eruption can be partial or complete. Posterior teeth are more commonly involved. Both primary and permanent teeth may be affected. Involved permanent teeth tend to become ankylosed. The application of orthodontic forces leads to ankylosis. The involvement may be unilateral or bilateral. The condition shows an absence of affected family members. Although several findings of Proffit and Vig's article can still be considered valid, the hereditary aspect has been revised. Indeed, many recently published studies have found an important familial-based aspect for this condition.

Hanisch et al. in their review [16] found that 84.1% of the patients of their sample had family members that reported having had PFE. In fact, patients with PFE revealed a mutation in the parathyroid hormone 1 receptor gene (*PTH1R*) that is transmitted by autosomal dominant inheritance [14]. This mutation is transmitted with an incomplete penetrance [21]. This gene encodes a member of the G-protein coupled receptor, and it is a receptor for parathyroid hormone (PTH). Normally, the PTH receptor is expressed in bone tissue on the surface of the osteoblast. A key function of PTH is the regulation of calcium metabolism [24]. After the activation of the receptor, the osteoclasts are stimulated to increase bone resorption, allowing tooth eruption. Other variants in *PTH1R* have also been associated with Jansen chondrodysplasia and Ollier enchondromatosis. These conditions are characterized by abnormal skeletal development [25]. PFE is now the fifth disease to be associated with mutations in the *PTH1R* gene [6]. Grippaudo et al. have hypothesized that the PFE phenotype could also be the result of a dose-dependent inactivation of *PTH1R* [2]. Considering the heritability of this condition, it is important to do an evaluation of the patient's family history through interviews. After that, it is helpful to analyze the *PTH1R* gene before planning the treatment. In 2021, Grippaudo et al. [10], through saliva samples, examined a cohort of patients that demonstrated clinical signs of PFE. DNA was extracted from saliva and subjected to PCR and sequencing. Some of the patients analyzed were genetically identified as carriers of variants of the *PTH1R* gene, while in others no variants were found. Through molecular analysis, they found 14 different variants. To be more specific, there were nine exonic *PTH1R* variants that had different effects on the protein structure. Above these there were a nonsense variant, a frameshift variant and missense variants. In patients with *PTH1R* variants that alter the protein structure, they found that the open bite is more severe and that Type 1 PFE is more frequently associated with a bilateral manifestation. On the other hand, not all the patients with an intronic variant had typical PFE. Other patients that did not demonstrate the presence of a *PTH1R* variant showed a less defined phenotype, sometimes limited to the involvement of a single tooth when compared to *PTH1R*-positive patients. According to this study, the typical traits of PFE are more often present in patients with pathogenic variants of the *PTH1R* gene. In addition, a patient who has signs of PFE may not have variants of the *PTH1R* gene. Furthermore, in their functional analysis of *PTH1R* variants [19], Izumida et al. showed that amino acid substitutions found in *PTH1R* from a patient with PFE lowered the responsiveness of the cells to PTH. These differences might have effects on the functions of osteoblasts and osteocytes. In fact, as said before, alterations in the balance between the resorptive and the appositional processes during the eruption are the putative factors underlying the development of PFE.

In addition to the clinical features of the PFE exposed by Proffit, subsequent articles reported that in patients with this condition, if an anterior tooth is affected, the posterior teeth are also affected; affected teeth resorb the alveolar bone coronal but do not erupt totally or erupt incomplete [23]; the growth of the alveolar process is impaired in the affected areas (in fact, the affected teeth appear at the base of a large vertical defect) [6]; a severe lateral open bite, unilateral or bilateral, is present [16]; and the affected molars show roots with dilacerations and truncation [17].

Regarding the possible treatment options for PFE, it is important to highlight that a dental element with PFE, if subjected to an orthodontic force, becomes ankylosed before achieving occlusion [12,13,26]. Considering this, treatment options are extremely limited. Before starting a treatment on these elements, it is important to wait until the end of the vertical growth of the patient. The treatment may be different considering the severity of the non-eruption. In particular, in patients that show a mild severity, the best option is a conservative restoration, for example, through onlays or crowns in order to close the open bite [15]. Instead, when the case is moderately severe, treatment options may include extraction or surgical removal of the teeth and subsequent implantation or orthodontic space closure. Another option is the segmental osteotomy to place in occlusion the element; in this case, all the segments involved are repositioned. Roulias et al. stated that when more than one tooth is affected, this type of treatment increases the chance of success [27]. If this is not possible, often a removable prosthesis is the only solution.

Table 1. Lists of the articles reviewed, with the subject of their main findings, type of article, and sample size. (Letter U = Unspecified).

Article	Epidemiology	Genotype	Phenotype	Treatment	Type of Article	Sample Size
Decker et al. (2008) [14]		✓	✓		Clinical research	15
Frazier-Bowers (2010) [24]		✓	✓		Clinical research	12
Stellzig-Eisenhauer et al. (2013) [6]	✓	✓			Clinical research	15
Frazier-Bowers et al. (2014) [21]		✓	✓		Clinical study	54
Milani et al. (2014) [15]	✓		✓	✓	Review	U
Pilz et al. (2014) [23]		✓	✓		Clinical research	36
Hanisch et al. (2018) [16]	✓	✓	✓	✓	Systematic review	314
Grippaudo et al. (2018) [2]		✓	✓		Clinical research	29
Izumida et al. (2020) [19]		✓			Clinical research	U
Tokavanich et al. (2020) [17]	✓	✓			In vivo animal study	U
Rizzo et al. (2020) [18]				✓	Review	U
Grippaudo et al. (2021) [10]	✓	✓	✓		Clinical research	38

5. Conclusions

To summarize, most of the analyzed articles agree on the importance of a differential diagnosis between PFE and other possible mechanisms, such as MFE or ankylosis [18], when a failure in a tooth eruption is observed, in the absence of systemic disorders. Considering the relevance of the genetic aspects that were exposed in this review, a *PTH1R* screening can be helpful to understand the reason of the non-eruption in order to choose the best treatment prior to any orthodontic treatment to avoid the ankylosis and avoid unnecessary and long-lasting therapies for patients that result in failure and expose them to iatrogenic damage. On the other hand, the research underlines a lack of information about treatment options: further studies are needed to assess which is the best way to treat PFE patients. Thus far, every treatment plan must be evaluated individually.

Author Contributions: Conceptualization: L.T. and G.G.; methodology: A.D.S.; validation: R.V.; formal analysis: R.V.; investigation: F.S. and C.S.; data curation: A.D.S.; writing—original draft preparation: F.S.; writing—review and editing: C.S.; visualization: R.V.; supervision: L.T. and G.G.; project administration: A.D.S. All authors have read and agreed to the published version of the manuscript.

Funding: This research received no external funding.

Institutional Review Board Statement: Not applicable.

Informed Consent Statement: Not applicable.

Data Availability Statement: Not applicable.

Conflicts of Interest: The authors declare no conflict of interest.

References

1. Schour, I.; Massler, M. Studies In Tooth Development: The Growth Pattern Of Human Teeth Part II. *J. Am. Dent. Assoc.* **1940**, *27*, 1918–1931. [CrossRef]
2. Grippaudo, C.; Cafiero, C.; D'Apolito, I.; Ricci, B.; Frazier-Bowers, S.A. Primary Failure of Eruption: Clinical and Genetic Findings in the Mixed Dentition. *Angle Orthod.* **2018**, *88*, 275–282. [CrossRef] [PubMed]
3. Wise, G.E.; King, G.J. Mechanisms of Tooth Eruption and Orthodontic Tooth Movement. *J. Dent. Res.* **2008**, *87*, 414–434. [CrossRef] [PubMed]
4. Ono, W.; Sakagami, N.; Nishimori, S.; Ono, N.; Kronenberg, H.M. Parathyroid Hormone Receptor Signalling in Osterix-Expressing Mesenchymal Progenitors Is Essential for Tooth Root Formation. *Nat. Commun.* **2016**, *7*, 11277. [CrossRef]
5. Marks, S.C.; Cahill, D.R.; Wise, G.E. The Cytology of the Dental Follicle and Adjacent Alveolar Bone during Tooth Eruption in the Dog. *Am. J. Anat.* **1983**, *168*, 277–289. [CrossRef] [PubMed]
6. Stellzig-Eisenhauer, A.; Decker, E.; Meyer-Marcotty, P.; Rau, C.; Fiebig, B.S.; Kress, W.; Saar, K.; Rüschendorf, F.; Hubner, N.; Grimm, T.; et al. Primary failure of eruption (PFE). Clinical and molecular genetics analysis. *Orthod. Fr.* **2013**, *84*, 241–250. [CrossRef]
7. Impellizzeri, A.; Palaia, G.; Horodynski, M.; Pergolini, D.; Vernucci, R.A.; Romeo, U.; Galluccio, G. Co2 laser for surgical exposure of impacted palatally canines. *Dent. Cadmos* **2020**, *88*, 122–126. [CrossRef]
8. Raghoebar, G.M.; Boering, G.; Vissink, A.; Stegenga, B. Eruption Disturbances of Permanent Molars: A Review. *J. Oral Pathol. Med. Off. Publ. Int. Assoc. Oral Pathol. Am. Acad. Oral Pathol.* **1991**, *20*, 159–166. [CrossRef]
9. Alligri, A.; Putrino, A.; Cassetta, M.; Silvestri, A.; Barbato, E.; Galluccio, G. The Mandibular Permanent Second Molars and Their Risk of Impaction: A Retrospective Study. *Eur. J. Paediatr. Dent. Off. J. Eur. Acad. Paediatr. Dent.* **2015**, *16*, 246–250.
10. Grippaudo, C.; D'Apolito, I.; Cafiero, C.; Re, A.; Chiurazzi, P.; Frazier-Bowers, S.A. Validating Clinical Characteristic of Primary Failure of Eruption (PFE) Associated with PTH1R Variants. *Prog. Orthod.* **2021**, *22*, 43. [CrossRef]
11. Raghoebar, G.M.; Boering, G.; Vissink, A. Clinical, Radiographic and Histological Characteristics of Secondary Retention of Permanent Molars. *J. Dent.* **1991**, *19*, 164–170. [CrossRef]
12. Proffit, W.R.; Vig, K.W. Primary Failure of Eruption: A Possible Cause of Posterior Open-Bite. *Am. J. Orthod.* **1981**, *80*, 173–190. [CrossRef]
13. Frazier-Bowers, S.A.; Puranik, C.P.; Mahaney, M.C. The Etiology of Eruption Disorders—Further Evidence of a "Genetic Paradigm". *Semin. Orthod.* **2010**, *16*, 180–185. [CrossRef] [PubMed]
14. Decker, E.; Stellzig-Eisenhauer, A.; Fiebig, B.S.; Rau, C.; Kress, W.; Saar, K.; Rüschendorf, F.; Hubner, N.; Grimm, T.; Weber, B.H.F. PTHR1 Loss-of-Function Mutations in Familial, Nonsyndromic Primary Failure of Tooth Eruption. *Am. J. Hum. Genet.* **2008**, *83*, 781–786. [CrossRef] [PubMed]
15. Milani, M.S.; Kuijpers, M.A.R. Primary failure of eruption: Diagnostics, treatment, casus and review of literature. *Ned. Tijdschr. Tandheelkd.* **2014**, *121*, 227–232. [CrossRef]

16. Hanisch, M.; Hanisch, L.; Kleinheinz, J.; Jung, S. Primary Failure of Eruption (PFE): A Systematic Review. *Head Face Med.* **2018**, *14*, 5. [CrossRef]
17. Tokavanich, N.; Gupta, A.; Nagata, M.; Takahashi, A.; Matsushita, Y.; Yatabe, M.; Ruellas, A.; Cevidanes, L.; Maki, K.; Yamaguchi, T.; et al. A Three-Dimensional Analysis of Primary Failure of Eruption in Humans and Mice. *Oral Dis.* **2020**, *26*, 391–400. [CrossRef]
18. Rizzo, M.; Colard, T.; Bocquet, E.; Leverd, C. Primary failure of eruption: Combined vision between paediatric dentist and orthodontist. *Orthod. Fr.* **2020**, *91*, 47–55. [CrossRef]
19. Izumida, E.; Suzawa, T.; Miyamoto, Y.; Yamada, A.; Otsu, M.; Saito, T.; Yamaguchi, T.; Nishimura, K.; Ohtaka, M.; Nakanishi, M.; et al. Functional Analysis of PTH1R Variants Found in Primary Failure of Eruption. *J. Dent. Res.* **2020**, *99*, 429–436. [CrossRef]
20. Baccetti, T. Tooth Anomalies Associated with Failure of Eruption of First and Second Permanent Molars. *Am. J. Orthod. Dentofac. Orthop. Off. Publ. Am. Assoc. Orthod. Its Const. Soc. Am. Board Orthod.* **2000**, *118*, 608–610. [CrossRef]
21. Frazier-Bowers, S.A.; Hendricks, H.M.; Wright, J.T.; Lee, J.; Long, K.; Dibble, C.F.; Bencharit, S. Novel Mutations in PTH1R Associated with Primary Failure of Eruption and Osteoarthritis. *J. Dent. Res.* **2014**, *93*, 134–139. [CrossRef] [PubMed]
22. Calasso, S.; Cassetta, M.; Galluccio, G.; Barbato, E. Impacted lower second molars. *Dent. Cadmos* **2008**, *76*, 41–54.
23. Pilz, P.; Meyer-Marcotty, P.; Eigenthaler, M.; Roth, H.; Weber, B.H.F.; Stellzig-Eisenhauer, A. Differential Diagnosis of Primary Failure of Eruption (PFE) with and without Evidence of Pathogenic Mutations in the PTHR1 Gene. *J. Orofac. Orthop. Fortschr. Kieferorthop.* **2014**, *75*, 226–239. [CrossRef]
24. Frazier-Bowers, S.A.; Simmons, D.; Wright, J.T.; Proffit, W.R.; Ackerman, J.L. Primary Failure of Eruption and PTH1R: The Importance of a Genetic Diagnosis for Orthodontic Treatment Planning. *Am. J. Orthod. Dentofac. Orthop. Off. Publ. Am. Assoc. Orthod. Its Const. Soc. Am. Board Orthod.* **2010**, *137*, 160.e1–160.e7; discussion 160–161. [CrossRef] [PubMed]
25. Schipani, E.; Kruse, K.; Jüppner, H. A Constitutively Active Mutant PTH-PTHrP Receptor in Jansen-Type Metaphyseal Chondrodysplasia. *Science* **1995**, *268*, 98–100. [CrossRef]
26. O'Connell, A.C.; Torske, K.R. Primary Failure of Tooth EruptionA Unique Case. *Oral Surg. Oral Med. Oral Pathol. Oral Radiol. Endodontol.* **1999**, *87*, 714–720. [CrossRef]
27. Roulias, P.; Kalantzis, N.; Doukaki, D.; Pachiou, A.; Karamesinis, K.; Damanakis, G.; Gizani, S.; Tsolakis, A.I. Teeth Eruption Disorders: A Critical Review. *Children* **2022**, *9*, 771. [CrossRef]

Review

Could Periodontitis Aggravate Psoriasis?—An Update by Systematic Review

Juan José Meneu [1], Cecilia Fabiana Márquez-Arrico [2,3,*], Francisco Javier Silvestre [2,3] and Javier Silvestre-Rangil [3]

[1] Department of Dentistry, Faculty of Health Sciences, European University of Valencia, 46010 Valencia, Spain
[2] Unit of Stomatology, Dr. Peset University Hospital, 46017 Valencia, Spain
[3] Faculty of Medicine and Dentistry, University of Valencia, 46010 Valencia, Spain
* Correspondence: dra.cecilia.marquez@gmail.com; Tel.: +34-963-188-787

Abstract: (1) Background: Psoriasis is a chronic and inflammatory systemic disease that has been associated with periodontal pathologies, specifically periodontitis. The aim of this research is to answer the following question: Could periodontitis aggravate psoriasis? (2) Methods: We carried out a systematic review following the PRISMA guide using PubMed, Embase, Scopus, and WOS; (3) Results: A total of 111 studies were identified in the databases and 11 were obtained after screening. The selection included nine case–control studies, one cross-sectional study, and one cohort study. Most of the publications report an increase in bleeding on probing and the presence of periodontal pockets in patients with psoriasis, confirming that inflammation caused by periodontitis can contribute to systemic inflammation worsening psoriasis. To summarize, the scientific literature indicates that local periodontal inflammation could aggravate psoriasis.

Keywords: psoriasis; periodontitis; inflammatory disease; periodontal disease; risk factors for psoriasis

Citation: Meneu, J.J.; Márquez-Arrico, C.F.; Silvestre, F.J.; Silvestre-Rangil, J. Could Periodontitis Aggravate Psoriasis?—An Update by Systematic Review. *Oral* **2023**, *3*, 57–66. https://doi.org/10.3390/oral3010006

Academic Editors: Giuseppina Campisi and Vera Panzarella

Received: 12 December 2022
Revised: 7 January 2023
Accepted: 10 January 2023
Published: 16 January 2023

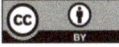

Copyright: © 2023 by the authors. Licensee MDPI, Basel, Switzerland. This article is an open access article distributed under the terms and conditions of the Creative Commons Attribution (CC BY) license (https:// creativecommons.org/licenses/by/ 4.0/).

1. Introduction

Psoriasis is a chronic, immune-mediated inflammatory skin disease, characterized by red and scaly plaques occurring more frequently on the elbows, knees, scalp, and lower back [1]. Worldwide, in 2017, an estimated 29.5 million adults had psoriasis, corresponding to a physician-diagnosed lifetime prevalence of 0.59% of the adult population [1]. Plaque psoriasis is the most frequent type, representing more than 80% of psoriasis cases [2]. The pathogenesis of plaque psoriasis consists of a feed-forward mechanism of inflammation involving primarily the T-helper cell type 17 (TH17) pathway [2]. In the past, psoriasis was considered a disease that was limited to the skin and was treated with topical agents or phototherapy. With recent advances, research has focused on clarifying the roles of specific proinflammatory cytokines that contribute to the disease's pathogenesis [3].

Psoriasis is a visible skin disease, and therefore relationships with other people can be disturbed. Many patients encounter prejudice and rejection and feel that their attractiveness is diminished. Therapy and skin care are time-consuming, so psoriasis patients may be limited in their work, leisure time, and freedom of movement due to physical symptoms [1,4]. Apart from comorbidities [5], people with psoriasis not only have to cope with physical limitations but also with severe psychological burdens such as depression, anxiety, and suicidal thoughts [1,4].

Guideline-indicated therapeutic options involve topical treatments, phototherapy, and systemic therapies which encompass both oral treatments and injectable biologics. Eighty per cent of patients with psoriasis have mild-to-moderate forms of psoriasis and can be treated exclusively with topical agents such as corticosteroids and vitamin D analogs. Phototherapy and systemic agents are recommended for patients with moderate-to-severe psoriasis, where the extent of the disease makes topical therapy of all lesions impractical [6].

Recently, psoriasis has been related to other chronic inflammatory conditions, such as periodontitis. Accumulated epidemiologic, genetic, and pathogenetic evidence indicates that psoriasis is associated with this condition [7]. The American Academy of Periodontics defines periodontal disease as an inflammation of the supporting tissues of the tooth [8]. It is a progressive destruction process that leads to the loss of the supporting bone of the tooth and its periodontal ligament [9]. The prevalence of periodontitis is reported to vary from 20% to 50% around the world. Additionally, periodontitis is one of the major causes of tooth loss, which can undermine function, aesthetics, self-confidence, and quality of life [10].

Periodontitis is a chronic inflammatory condition provoked by a bacterial infection that activates the host immune response [10–16]. Psoriasis could cause periodontal lesions and sometimes white plaque and erythema lesions on the oral mucosa and palate [11,16]. This disease is an inflammatory condition considered a result of the complex interaction between the oral microbial community and the host response, modified by genetics and environmental factors. In recent decades, there has been increasing evidence supporting a strong relationship between periodontitis and systemic conditions. These conditions include cardiovascular diseases, metabolic syndrome, obesity, rheumatoid arthritis, polycystic ovary syndrome, and adverse outcomes during pregnancy [11–13].

Since psoriasis and periodontitis have similar pathogenic mechanisms and associated conditions in common, there has been a renewed interest in research into possible links between these diseases. The current hypothesis of common etiopathogenic processes between the conditions comprises several possible mechanisms, such as amplified inflammatory response and T-cell activation and a lower concentration of salivary IgA and lysozymes [11]. Some studies have already indicated that patients with psoriasis have a significantly elevated risk of periodontitis compared with controls without psoriasis [14–20]. This was especially observed in patients with severe psoriasis [21]. In addition, a meta-analysis reported that patients with periodontitis have a significantly increased risk of psoriasis [22]. Therefore, the aim of this study was to establish if periodontitis could aggravate psoriasis and if psoriasis patients had more risk of developing periodontal disease or presenting worse periodontal status.

2. Materials and Methods

We carried out a systematic review following the PRISMA guide (Preferred Reporting Items for Systematic Reviews and Meta-analyses), and the PRISMA check list is available as Supplementary Materials [23]. We built an evidence-based research method for incorporating a PECO question model (PECO: Participants, Exposure, Control and Outcomes). The focused question was: Could periodontitis aggravate psoriasis? Patients (P): patients with psoriasis; Exposure (E): exposition to periodontitis; Control (C): periodontal healthy patients. Outcome (O): periodontal and clinical parameters. It was intended to establish if periodontitis can be considered a risk cofactor for aggravating periodontal problems in patients in comparison with healthy patients. The chronic inflammation that exists in periodontitis could cause higher vulnerability to developing more clinical manifestations of psoriasis.

2.1. Search Strategy

To carry out the systematic review we used the following databases: PubMed (National Library of Medicine, Washington, DC, USA), Embase, Scopus (Elsevier B.V., Amsterdam, The Netherlands), and Web of Science Core Collection. The keywords employed were: periodontitis, psoriasis, inflammation, and inflammatory disorder. The search strategy was performed using MeSH terms. To facilitate the reproducibility of the search strategy, a QR code was generated for each database used (Figure 1). This systematic review was registered in PROSPERO, the international prospective register of systematic reviews, with the following registration code: CRD42021261141.

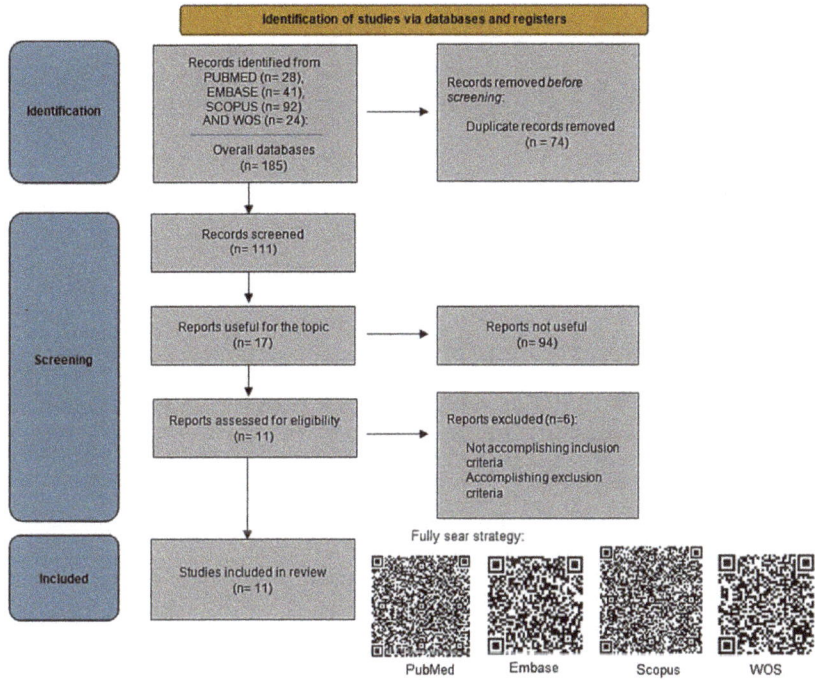

Figure 1. Flow chart following the PRISMA guide [23].

2.2. Selection of Articles and Eligibility Criteria

The inclusion criteria were: original research articles reporting longitudinal studies, cross-sectional studies, clinical trials, cohort studies, or case–control studies in the previous 5 years. Besides, the sample size included was research with 30 or more individuals and articles with quality score of 4 or higher. The exclusion criteria were: topic reviews, case reports, and low quality articles. After conducting a bibliographic search, duplicate articles were removed. Moreover, studies that were not deemed useful for the topic were excluded. Finally, those articles which did not meet the inclusion criteria were not considered for this systematic review. Thus, a selection of articles was established to answer the PECO question (Figure 1).

2.3. Quality Control of Articles

The Newcastle–Ottawa scale for quality control was used. This scale checks the selection of the study groups, the comparability of the groups, and the outcomes (exposure for case–control studies). It is a "gold standard" system that assesses these 3 features, with each comprising several items depending on the type of publication: case–control study (Table 1), cross-sectional study (Table 2), and cohort study (Table 3).

Table 1. Newcastle–Ottawa scale for case–control study.

Author, Year	Selection Items				Comparability Item	Exposure Items			Total
	1	2	3	4	5	6	7	8	
Sezer et al., 2016			*	*	*	*	*		6/9
Painsi et al., 2017				*	*	*	*		4/9
Sarac et al., 2017		*	*	*	*	*	*		6/9
Woeste et al., 2019	*	*	*	*	*	*			6/9
Macklis et al., 2019	*	*	*		*	*			5/9
Mendes et al., 2019	*	*	*	*	*	*			6/9
Barros et al., 2020	*			*	*	*	*		5/9
Belstrøm et al., 2020	*				*	*	*		4/9
Skutnik-Radziszewska et al., 2020	*	*			*	*	*		5/9

Selection: 1: Is the case definition adequate? (1 point); 2: Representativeness of the cases (1 point); 3: Selection of controls (1 point); 4: Definition of controls (1 point); Comparability: 5: Comparability of cases and controls on the basis of the design (1 point) or/and analysis (1 point); Exposure: 6: Ascertainment of exposure (1 point); 7: Same method of ascertainment for cases and controls (1 point); 8: Non-response rate (1 point). *: Corresponds to 1 point from total score when the research adequately meets the item.

Table 2. Newcastle-Ottawa scale for cross-sectional study.

Author, Year	Selection Items				Comparability Item	Outcome Items		Total
	1	2	3	4	5	6	7	
Ligia et al., 2019	*			**	*	**		6/9

Selection: 1: Representativeness of the sample (1 point); 2: Sample size (1 point); 3: Non-respondents (1 point); 4: Ascertainment of exposure (2 points); Comparability: 5: Subjects in different outcomes are comparable, based on the study design or analysis, and confounding factors are controlled (1 point); Outcome: 6: Assessment of the outcome (2 points); 7: Statistical test (1 point). *: Corresponds to 1 point from total score when the research adequately meets the item. **: 2 points.

Table 3. Newcastle-Ottawa Scale for cohort study.

Author, Year	Selection Items				Comparability Item	Outcome Items			Total
	1	2	3	4	5	6	7	8	
Egeberg et al., 2017	*	*	*		**	*	*		7/9

Selection: 1: Representativeness of the exposed cohort (1 point); 2: Selection of the non-exposed cohort (1 point); 3: Ascertainment of exposure (1 point); 4: Demonstration that outcome of interest was not present at start of study (1 point); Comparability: 5: Comparability of cohorts on the basis of the design or analysis (2 points); Outcome: 6: Assessment of outcome (1 point); 7: Was follow up long enough for outcomes to occur (1 point); 8: Adequacy of follow up of cohorts (1 point). *: Corresponds to 1 point from total score when the research adequately meets the item. **: 2 points.

3. Results

In this systematic review, a total of 111 studies were identified in the databases, and 11 were obtained after screening (Figure 1). The selection included nine case–control studies, one cross-sectional study, and one cohort study. The general characteristics of the studies analyzed in this review are presented in Table 4. All the articles used large samples of between 71 and 5,470,428 individuals. Regarding the case–control studies, these mainly compared the results of periodontal tests and epidemiological indexes (prevalence and incidence) between a group exposed to psoriasis and a control group. In the cross-sectional study, the periodontal status of the sample was analyzed. In the cohort study, the different periodontal states of different groups were compared, including psoriasis patient groups and control groups. Most of the publications report an increase in bleeding on probing and the presence of periodontal pockets in patients with psoriasis and indicate that local periodontal inflammation could aggravate psoriasis.

Table 4. General characteristics of the studies analysed in this review.

Author, Year	Type of Study	Sample Size	Periodontal Evaluation	Conclusions
Sezer et al., 2016	Case–control	100 cases 20 controls	PI, PD, CAL, and BOP%	There were no differences between periodontitis (systemically healthy-chronic periodontitis, psoriasis-chronic periodontitis, psoriatic arthritis-chronic periodontitis) groups
Painsi et al., 2017	Case–control	209 cases 91 controls	Data from patient who underwent an inflammatory focus screening, including a dental check up	Higher periodontitis prevalence in psoriasis patients compared with chronic spontaneous urticaria (OR = 3.76; 95% CI 1.60–10.27; p = 0.001)
Sarac et al., 2017	Case–control	76 cases 76 controls	CPITN	In the psoriasis group, there were higher values in CPITN
Woeste et al., 2019	Case–control	100 cases 101 controls	BOP, CPITN, and dental parameters according to the DMFTI	The author found higher values in BOP and CPITN in psoriasis group. There were no differences for DMFTI. Periodontitis could aggravate psoriasis simptosms.
Macklis et al., 2019	Case–control	100 cases 165 controls	Validated WHO survey for adult oral hygiene practices including gingivitis and periodontitis signs	Patients who reported poor or very poor gum health showed more symptoms of severe psoriasis. Periodontitis could aggravate psoriasis simptosms.
Mendes et al., 2019	Case–control	397 cases 325 controls	PI, PD, CAL, and BOP	Psoriasis patients had higher PI, PD, BOP, and CAL values. Psoriasis individuals showed more probability of suffering periodontitis when compared with controls (OR = 1.72; 95% CI 1.28–2.32; p < 0.001).
Barros et al., 2020	Case–control	69 cases 74 controls	PI, PD, CAL, BOP, and DMFTI	Psoriasis patients had lower PI values, higher CAL and DMFT values, and fewer teeth. More prevalence of severe and generalized periodontitis. Severe periodontitis can be considered a risk factor for psoriasis (OR = 3.7; 95% CI 1.5–9.0; p < 0.003). BOP was not significantly different.
Belstrøm et al., 2020	Case–control	85 cases 52 controls	PI, BOP, PD, and CAL	Patients with psoriasis had good periodontal health (regularly attending dental care). No differences in missing teeth, PD, or CAL. Relatively high percentages of BOP and PI. Lower salivary levels of NGAL and transferrin.
Skutnik-Radziszewska et al., 2020	Case–control	40 cases 40 controls	Dental status, DMFTI, PBI, and GI	There were no differences in the values of DMFTI, PBI, or GI

Table 4. Cont.

Author, Year	Type of Study	Sample Size	Periodontal Evaluation	Conclusions
Ligia et al., 2019	Cross-sectional	71 participants	PI, BOP, CAL, and PD	Periodontal disease was frequent in patients with psoriasis. Nevertheless, there was no statistically significant (small sample). No data for periodontal indexes.
Egeberg et al., 2017	Cohort	5,470,428 participants	Patients with periodontitis were identified by their first inpatient or outpatient (ambulatory) hospital diagnosis of periodontitis	Increased risk of periodontitis in mild psoriasis linebreak (IRR: 1.66; 95% CI 1.43–1.94; $p < 0.001$), severe psoriasis (IRR: 2.24; 95% CI 1.46–3.44; $p < 0.001$) and psoriatic arthritis (IRR: 3.48; 95% CI 2.46–4.92; $p < 0.001$). Periodontitis could agravate psoriasis simptosms.

Abbreviations: PI: plaque index; CAL: clinical attachment loss; BOP: bleeding on probing; PD: probing depth; GI: gingival index; CPITN: community periodontal index of treatment needs; DMFTI: decayed, missing, and filled teeth index; D: decayed teeth; M: missing teeth; FT: filled teeth; PBI: papilla bleeding index; IRR: incidence rate ratio.

3.1. Periodontal Parameters

The periodontal parameters used in most of the investigations were probing depth (PD) [18,19,24–26], clinical attachment loss (CAL) [18,19,24–26], and the community periodontal index of treatment need (CPITN) (15,16). All of these indices are indicative of the stage of periodontitis according to the new classification of 2017 [27]. PD had higher values in one study [18], but in the others that analyzed it there were no differences between cases and controls [19,24–26]. CAL had higher values in some of the studies reviewed [18,19] but not in others [24–26]. There were significant differences in CPITN in the two studies involving it [15,16]. In addition, plaque index (PI) was used to assess the oral hygiene of some patients [18,19,24–26], with most studies finding no differences in this measure between cases and controls.

On the other hand, other authors have used some less frequent indexes, such as bleeding on probing (BOP) [16,18,19,24–26]; the decayed, missing, and filled teeth index (DMFTI) [16,19,28]; the papilla bleeding index (PBI) [28]; and the gingival index (GI) [28] (Table 4).

3.2. Epidemiological Parameters

Likewise, it is especially important to mention the epidemiological factors identified in this review. Some of the studies used prevalence indicators [14,18,19] while other publications used incidence rates [20]. Thus, the prevalence of periodontitis was 23.9–46.1% in psoriasis patients compared with 7.7–33.1% in healthy controls [14,18]. An OR of between 1.72 (95% CI 1.28–2.32; $p < 0.001$) [18] and 3.76 (95% CI 1.60–10.27; $p = 0.001$) [14] was found for the risk of psoriasis patients suffering periodontitis. Regarding the incidence of periodontitis in the cohort study [20], the authors found significant differences between cases and controls. The incidence rate ratio (IRR) in mild psoriasis was 1.66 (95% CI 1.43–1.94; $p < 0.001$), 2.24 (95% CI 1.46–3.44; $p < 0.001$) in psoriatic arthritis, and 3.48 (95% CI 2.46–4.92; $p < 0.001$) in severe psoriasis. Finally, Macklis [17] used a validated WHO survey to establish the state of gums in adult patients with psoriasis compared with healthy controls, and it was observed that psoriasis patients who considered their gum health to be poor or very poor had significantly more severe psoriasis symptoms.

4. Discussion

This systematic review has given our PECO question an affirmative answer with periodontitis being a disease that could aggravate the clinical manifestations of psoriasis. Patients with psoriasis present an increase in proinflammatory cytokines that leads to a bidirectional association between both pathologies [14–20,24–26,28]. This topic has attracted interest because of the effects that both diseases have on patients and because of the large number of people who suffer from both of them. These two conditions share several common immunologic, micro-biological, and environmental pathogenetic factors. Although the etiopathogenesis is not fully understood, it is proposed that the environmental factors modify the diversity of the local microbiome and produce dysbiosis. Altogether, these factors lead to T-cell activation and cytokine production [7], which starts the inflammatory process. Thus, there has been increasing attention in establishing if psoriasis and periodontitis have a relationship.

In two previous similar studies it was determined that psoriasis patients had higher chances of suffering from periodontitis. Qiao et al. [21] carried out a meta-analysis of eight articles, finding significant differences in BOP, PD, CAL, and remaining and missing teeth, as well as in the level of alveolar bone loss. There were no differences in PI and GI. The authors elucidated that psoriasis patients suffer from worse periodontal health compared with non-psoriasis subjects, and, despite a more detailed investigation being needed, it was concluded that the confounding factors should be taken into much more consideration. Moreover, it was stated that there were not enough studies to establish solid conclusions for some indexes and that more papers should undertake adequate quality meta-analysis. Zhang et al. [11] performed a systematic review, concluding that psoriasis and periodontitis were bidirectionally related, but the authors mention that there was high heterogeneity among the papers and a higher number of articles was needed. Zang et al. [11] also report that the role of confounding factors such as age, gender, or systemic conditions should be highlighted. Additionally, establishing precise and common criteria for the diagnosis of periodontitis was deemed critical. Regarding the present paper, there were three studies that did not find any differences between the psoriasis patients and the control groups [25,26,28]. Ligia et al. (24) also show no statistical significance between groups, although periodontitis was more frequent in psoriasis patients. The remaining seven articles [13–19] gathered significant evidence that patients with psoriasis were more susceptible to suffering periodontal disease. These articles [14–20] used epidemiological indexes (prevalence [14,18,19] and incidence [20]), periodontal indexes [15,16,18,19], and questionnaires [17]. In several studies [13,17,18], it was found that there was a higher prevalence of periodontitis in psoriasis patients with an OR (95% CI) of between 1.72 (1.28–2.32, $p < 0.001$) [18] and 3.76 (1.60–10.27, $p = 0.001$) [14]. Eberg et al.'s cohort study [20] has to be highlighted as the initial sample was all individuals aged 18 or over from Denmark, with a final sample was composed of 5,470,428 individuals. Their results show through the IRR that there is an increased risk of periodontitis in mild psoriasis (IRR: 1.66; 95% CI 1.43–1.94; $p < 0.001$), severe psoriasis (IRR: 2.24; 95% CI 1.46–3.44; $p < 0.001$), and psoriatic arthritis (IRR: 3.48; 95% CI 2.46–4.92; $p < 0.001$).

However, the results are not as clear for the PD measure with four out of five articles not finding any differences [19,24–26]. For the CAL measure, three out of five papers found no differences between cases and controls [24–26]. Furthermore, all of the studies that analyzed PI did not find any differences [18,19,24–26]. Regarding prevalence, three out of three studies showed significant differences [14,18,19]. All of this may indicate that psoriasis can be a risk factor for developing periodontal disease. Nevertheless, the diagnosis of periodontitis in these three publications was different. While Painsi et al. [14] used registers to identify periodontal disease patients, Mendes et al. [18] employed interproximal CAL and/or PD and Barros et al. [19] only used the CAL measure in interproximal sites. The different diagnosis methods in the studies increases the heterogeneity of the results and the subsequent conclusions. For further studies, there should be criteria for always establishing the same method of diagnosis since without this, it is difficult to compare and generalize results, especially in relation to registers. Although it is a good method for large studies, it reduces their precision. Thus, a goal for this line of research would be having a common diagnosis for both periodontitis and psoriasis.

In addition, there is the question of confounding factors, with age, gender, or systemic conditions having been mentioned already. However, there may be other factors that have the capacity to modify the results. Socioeconomic status is likely to alter periodontitis outcomes, so patients with less access to healthcare or healthy conditions are more likely to have worse outcomes. Another confounding factor is the presence of plaque, as there will not be the same outcomes for people with poor hygiene vs. people with good oral care. There have been articles involved in some systematic reviews with very high PI values, and these values are going to change the results because the periodontium is not going to react in the same way to good hygiene as it does to poor hygiene. Both diseases have been shown to cause inflammatory changes in the form of increased cytokine values [14–16,19,20,24–26]. Since they are essential in the pathogenesis and progression of periodontitis and psoriasis, it can be speculated that increased cytokine values may favor the development of periodontitis [14–16,18,26]. This altered state would render the individual susceptible to developing inflammatory diseases. Therefore, it has been shown that if periodontal disease is treated, the psoriasis condition improves [29,30]. In addition, systemic psoriasis therapy could lead to better periodontal parameters [29–31].

An association between psoriasis and periodontitis has been shown, and increased concentrations of proinflammatory cytokines such as TNF-α and IL-1β have been found in saliva from patients with psoriasis [3,30–32]. Activated TH17 cells producing IL-17 are key pathogenic players in psoriasis, and bacterial infection, including infection with *P. gingivalis*, may also activate TH17 cells. This bacterial infection can activate inflammatory pathways, promoting secretion of interleukins and increasing the clinical manifestations of psoriasis by contributing to systemic inflammation. Moreover, activated TH17 cells have been found in periodontal lesions and in mild psoriasis, and increased IL-17 levels have been demonstrated in crevicular fluid from patients with mild psoriasis [2,3,30–32]. These findings show that TH17 hyperactivation could be a pathway that connects both pathologies, sharing pathophysiological mechanisms present in psoriasis and periodontitis [2,3,7,17–19,31–33].

However, there is some heterogeneity in the results of recent articles on this topic, which could be because the investigations used different diagnosis methods for periodontitis. Prospective and more detailed research is required to obtain more evidence. In any case, this manuscript has carried out a review following the PRISMA guidelines [23] and using quality scales with a thorough protocol developed by three researches with experience in this field. Moreover, this publication covers the most recent articles on the subject and has incorporated the most cited papers on the relationship between periodontitis and psoriasis.

5. Conclusions

The scientific literature available up to now affirms that periodontitis could aggravate the clinical manifestations of psoriasis. A bidirectional association between both pathologies is proposed: On the one hand, patients with psoriasis typically present oral lesions that make them more at risk of developing periodontal diseases [1,4,6,11,16], and on the other hand, periodontitis in patients with psoriasis may increase the poll of proinflammatory cytokines and in this way aggravate the clinical manifestations of psoriasis [14–20,24–26,28,31,32]. Clearly, the role of the dentist is of great importance, since a dental examination can identify the presence of periodontitis and provide treatment to patients. This treatment can improve the systemic inflammatory process and improve the evolution of psoriasis, so periodontal treatment would also improve the consequences of psoriasis. In addition, since the evidence points to periodontitis and psoriasis having a bidirectional relationship, dental practitioners should carry out a comprehensive dental checkup in these populations. Patients diagnosed with psoriasis could also undergo specific gum surveillance, since there is evidence that psoriasis may be a risk factor for periodontitis too.

Supplementary Materials: The following supporting information can be downloaded at: https://www.mdpi.com/article/10.3390/oral3010006/s1, The PRISMA check list.

Author Contributions: Conceptualization, J.J.M., C.F.M.-A., F.J.S. and J.S.-R.; methodology, J.J.M., C.F.M.-A., F.J.S. and J.S.-R.; formal analysis and investigation, J.J.M., C.F.M.-A., F.J.S. and J.S.-R.; resources, data curation, writing—original draft preparation, J.J.M., C.F.M.-A. and F.J.S.; writing—review and editing, J.J.M., C.F.M.-A., F.J.S. and J.S.-R.; visualization and supervision, F.J.S. and J.S.-R.; project administration, J.J.M., C.F.M.-A., F.J.S. and J.S.-R.; funding acquisition, C.F.M.-A. and F.J.S. All authors have read and agreed to the published version of the manuscript.

Funding: This research was funded by grant number 18/00854 from the Ministry of Science, Innovation, and Universities of Spain.

Institutional Review Board Statement: Not applicable.

Informed Consent Statement: Not applicable.

Data Availability Statement: Not applicable.

Acknowledgments: We thank the Ministry of Science, Innovation, and Universities for the grant received.

Conflicts of Interest: The authors declare no conflict of interest.

References

1. Parisi, R.; Iskandar, I.Y.K.; Kontopantelis, E.; Augustin, M.; Griffiths, C.E.M.; Ashcroft, D.M. National, regional, and worldwide epidemiology of psoriasis: Systematic analysis and modelling study. *BMJ* **2020**, *369*, m1590. [CrossRef] [PubMed]
2. Armstrong, A.W.; Read, C. Pathophysiology, Clinical Presentation, and Treatment of Psoriasis: A Review. *JAMA* **2020**, *323*, 1945–1960. [CrossRef] [PubMed]
3. Korman, N.J. Management of psoriasis as a systemic disease: What is the evidence? *Br. J. Dermatol.* **2020**, *182*, 840–848. [CrossRef]
4. Bangemann, K.; Schulz, W.; Wohlleben, J.; Weyergraf, A.; Snitjer, I.; Werfel, T.; Schmid-Ott, G.; Böhm, D. Depression und Angststörung bei Psoriasispatienten: Schutz- und Risikofaktoren. *Hautarzt* **2014**, *65*, 1056–1061. [CrossRef] [PubMed]
5. Gerdes, S.; Mrowietz, U. Komorbiditäten und psoriasis: Konsequenzen für die praxis. *Hautarzt* **2012**, *63*, 202–213. [CrossRef]
6. Murage, M.J.; Kern, D.M.; Chang, L.; Sonawane, K.; Malatestinic, W.N.; Quimbo, R.A.; Feldman, S.R.; Muram, T.M.; Araujo, A.B. Treatment patterns among patients with psoriasis using a large national payer database in the United States: A retrospective study. *J. Med. Econ.* **2018**, *22*, 53–62. [CrossRef]
7. Dalmády, S.; Kemény, L.; Antal, M.; Gyulai, R. Periodontitis: A newly identified comorbidity in psoriasis and psoriatic arthritis. *Expert Rev. Clin. Immunol.* **2019**, *16*, 101–108. [CrossRef] [PubMed]
8. Anonymous. American Academy of Periodontology Task Force Report on the Update to the 1999 Classification of Periodontal Diseases and Conditions. *J. Periodontol.* **2015**, *86*, 835–838.
9. López Silva, M.C.; Diz-Iglesias, P.; Seoane-Romero, J.M.; Quintas, V.; Méndez-Brea, F.; Varela-Centelles, P. Actualización en medicina de familia: Patología periodontal. *Semergen* **2017**, *43*, 141–148. [CrossRef]
10. Nazir, M.; Al-Ansari, A.; Al-Khalifa, K.; Alhareky, M.; Gaffar, B.; Almas, K. Global Prevalence of Periodontal Disease and Lack of Its Surveillance. *Sci. World J.* **2020**, *2020*, 2146160. [CrossRef]
11. Zhang, X.; Gu, H.; Xie, S.; Su, Y. Periodontitis in patients with psoriasis: A systematic review and meta-analysis. *Oral Dis.* **2020**, *28*, 33–43. [CrossRef] [PubMed]
12. Martinez-Herrera, M.; Silvestre-Rangil, J.; Silvestre, F.J. Association between obesity and periodontal disease. A systematic review of epidemiological studies and controlled clinical trials. *Med. Oral Patol. Oral Cir. Bucal.* **2017**, *22*, e708–e715. [CrossRef] [PubMed]
13. Márquez-Arrico, C.F.; Silvestre-Rangil, J.; Gutiérrez-Castillo, L.; Martinez-Herrera, M.; Silvestre, F.J.; Rocha, M. Association between periodontal disease and polycystic ovary syndrome: A scoping review. *J. Oral. Res.* **2018**, *7*, 70–78.
14. Painsi, C.; Hirtenfelder, A.; Lange-Asschenfeldt, B.; Quehenberger, F.; Wolf, P. The Prevalence of Periodontitis Is Increased in Psoriasis and Linked to Its Inverse Subtype. *Ski. Pharmacol. Physiol.* **2017**, *30*, 324–328. [CrossRef]
15. Sarac, G.; Kapicioglu, Y.; Cayli, S.; Altas, A.; Yologlu, S. Is the periodontal status a risk factor for the development of psoriasis? *Niger. J. Clin. Pract.* **2017**, *20*, 474–478.
16. Woeste, S.; Graetz, C.; Gerdes, S.; Mrowietz, U. Oral Health in Patients with Psoriasis—A Prospective Study. *J. Investig. Dermatol.* **2019**, *139*, 1237–1244. [CrossRef]
17. Macklis, P.; Adams, K.M.; Li, D.; Krispinsky, A.; Bechtel, M.; Trinidad, J.; Kaffenberger, J.; Kumar, P.; Kaffenberger, B.H. The impacts of oral health symptoms, hygiene, and diet on the development and severity of psoriasis. *Dermatol. Online J.* **2019**, *25*, 16. [CrossRef]
18. Mendes, V.S.; Cota, L.O.M.; Costa, A.A.; Oliveira, A.M.S.D.; Costa, F.O. Periodontitis as another comorbidity associated with psoriasis: A case-control study. *J. Periodontol.* **2018**, *90*, 358–366. [CrossRef]
19. de Barros, F.C.; Sampaio, J.N.; Figueredo, C.M.d.S.; Carneiro, S.; Fischer, R.G. Higher Prevalence of Periodontitis and Decayed, Missing and Filled Teeth in Patients with Psoriasis. *Eur. J. Dent.* **2020**, *14*, 366–370. [CrossRef]

20. Egeberg, A.; Mallbris, L.; Gislason, G.; Hansen, P.; Mrowietz, U. Risk of periodontitis in patients with psoriasis and psoriatic arthritis. *J. Eur. Acad. Dermatol. Venereol.* **2016**, *31*, 288–293. [CrossRef]
21. Qiao, P.; Shi, Q.; Zhang, R.; Lingling, E.; Wang, P.; Wang, J.; Liu, H. Psoriasis Patients Suffer From Worse Periodontal Status—A Meta-Analysis. *Front. Med.* **2019**, *6*, 212. [CrossRef] [PubMed]
22. Ungprasert, P.; Wijarnpreecha, K.; Wetter, D. Periodontitis and risk of psoriasis: A systematic review and meta-analysis. *J. Eur. Acad. Dermatol. Venereol.* **2016**, *31*, 857–862. [CrossRef] [PubMed]
23. Page, M.J.; McKenzie, J.E.; Bossuyt, P.M.; Boutron, I.; Hoffmann, T.C.; Mulrow, C.D.; Shamseer, L.; Tetzlaff, J.; Akl, E.; Brennan, S.; et al. The PRISMA 2020 statement: An updated guideline for reporting systematic reviews. *BMJ* **2021**, *372*, n71. [CrossRef] [PubMed]
24. Ligia, M.G.; Leira, S.; Constanza, R.; Lorena, C.-M.; Rosa, B.M.; Nathaly, D.; Andrés, P.; Luis, A.C.; Consuelo, R.-S. Psoriasis Vulgaris: Relationship between Oral and Periodontal Conditions and Disease Severity. *Open Dermatol. J.* **2019**, *13*, 47–54. [CrossRef]
25. Belstrøm, D.; Eiberg, J.M.; Enevold, C.; Grande, M.A.; Jensen, C.A.J.; Skov, L.; Hansen, P.R. Salivary microbiota and inflammation-related proteins in patients with psoriasis. *Oral Dis.* **2020**, *26*, 677–687. [CrossRef]
26. Sezer, U.; Şenyurt, S.Z.; Gündoğar, H.; Erciyas, K.; Üstün, K.; Kimyon, G.; Kırtak, N.; Taysı, S.; Onat, A.M. Effect of Chronic Periodontitis on Oxidative Status in Patients with Psoriasis and Psoriatic Arthritis. *J. Periodontol.* **2016**, *87*, 557–565. [CrossRef]
27. Papapanou, P.N.; Sanz, M.; Buduneli, N.; Dietrich, T.; Feres, M.; Fine, D.H.; Flemmig, T.F.; Garcia, R.; Giannobile, W.V.; Graziani, F.; et al. Periodontitis: Consensus report of workgroup 2 of the 2017 World Workshop on the Classification of Periodontal and Peri-Implant Diseases and Conditions. *J. Periodontol.* **2018**, *89* (Suppl. S1), S173–S182. [CrossRef]
28. Skutnik-Radziszewska, A.; Maciejczyk, M.; Fejfer, K.; Krahel, J.; Flisiak, I.; Kołodziej, U.; Zalewska, A. Salivary Antioxidants and Oxidative Stress in Psoriatic Patients: Can Salivary Total Oxidant Status and Oxidative Status Index Be a Plaque Psoriasis Biomarker? *Oxid. Med. Cell. Longev.* **2020**, *2020*, 9086024. [CrossRef]
29. Ucan Yarkac, F.; Ogrum, A.; Gokturk, O. Effects of non-surgical periodontal therapy on inflammatory markers of psoriasis: A randomized controlled trial. *J. Clin. Periodontol.* **2020**, *26*, 193–201. [CrossRef]
30. Keller, J.; Lin, H. The effects of chronic periodontitis and its treatment on the subsequent risk of psoriasis. *Br. J. Dermatol.* **2012**, *167*, 1338–1344. [CrossRef]
31. Gokhale, S.R.; Padhye, A.M. Future prospects of systemic host modulatory agents in periodontal therapy. *Br. Dent. J.* **2013**, *214*, 467–471. [CrossRef] [PubMed]
32. Holmstrup, P.; Damgaard, C.; Olsen, I.; Klinge, B.; Flyvbjerg, A.; Nielsen, C.H.; Hansen, P.R. Comorbidity of periodontal disease: Two sides of the same coin? An introduction for the clinician. *J. Oral Microbiol.* **2017**, *9*, 1332710. [CrossRef] [PubMed]
33. Nijakowski, K.; Gruszczyński, D.; Kolasińska, J.; Kopała, D.; Surdacka, A. Periodontal Disease in Patients with Psoriasis: A Systematic Review. *Int. J. Environ. Res. Public Health* **2022**, *19*, 11302. [CrossRef] [PubMed]

Disclaimer/Publisher's Note: The statements, opinions and data contained in all publications are solely those of the individual author(s) and contributor(s) and not of MDPI and/or the editor(s). MDPI and/or the editor(s) disclaim responsibility for any injury to people or property resulting from any ideas, methods, instructions or products referred to in the content.

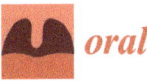

Article

Masticatory Functionality in Post-Acute-COVID-Syndrome (PACS) Patients with and without Sarcopenia

Bruno Davide Pugliese [1], Giovanna Garuti [1,*], Lucia Bergamini [1], Riccardo Karim Khamaisi [2], Giovanni Guaraldi [3], Ugo Consolo [1] and Pierantonio Bellini [1]

1. Unit of Dentistry & Oral-Maxillo-Facial Surgery, Department of Surgery, Medicine, Dentistry and Morphological Sciences, University of Modena and Reggio Emilia, 41125 Modena, Italy
2. Department of Engineering "Enzo Ferrari", University of Modena and Reggio Emilia, 41125 Modena, Italy
3. Infectious Diseases Unit, Department of Surgery, Medicine, Dentistry and Morphological Sciences, University of Modena and Reggio Emilia, 41125 Modena, Italy
* Correspondence: garuti.giovanna@gmail.com

Abstract: Musculoskeletal symptoms are common in both acute COVID-19 disease and post-acute sequelae (Post-Acute COVID Syndrome). The purpose of this study is to investigate whether there are reduced levels of masticatory function in patients with PACS (Post Acute COVID Syndrome) who suffer from sarcopenia, under the hypothesis that the latter may also involve the masticatory muscles. This study includes 23 patients hospitalized for COVID-19 between February 2020 and April 2021 and currently suffering from PACS. Among these PACS patients, 13/23 (56%) suffer from sarcopenia, 5/23 (22%) complain of asthenia but do not suffer from sarcopenia and the remaining 5/23 (22%) do not present muscle symptoms (non-asthenic non-sarcopenic). Oral health indices of all patients were collected. The masticatory strength was assessed with a gnathodynamometer based on piezoresistive sensors, and the masticatory effectiveness was measured by administering the "chewing gum mixing ability test" by having patients perform 20 masticatory cycles on a two-color chewing gum and analyzing the outcome through the ViewGum© software. Moreover, we gathered data with a hand grip test and gait speed test. The data collected in this study show that PACS sarcopenic patients have decreased masticatory effectiveness and strength compared to PACS asthenic non-sarcopenic patients and PACS non-asthenic non-sarcopenic patients.

Keywords: PACS (Post Acute COVID Syndrome); masticatory strength; sarcopenia

1. Introduction

ACE2 (angiotensin-converting enzyme) receptors are recognized as the prime target of SARS-CoV-2 (Severe Acute Respiratory Syndrome Coronavirus 2) [1], and the cellular infection causes the release of inflammatory cytokines [2–4]. As ACE2 receptors are present in multiple organs (lungs, trachea, intestines, skin, kidneys, pancreas, brain, heart and salivary glands [1,4,5]), the acute damage of COVID-19 (Coronavirus Disease 2019), caused by uncontrolled hyperinflammation, [3,6] is defined as multiorgan [7–9]. The World Health Organization has defined post-acute COVID-19 syndrome as long-term effects present for 3 months after a COVID-19 onset which cannot be explained by an alternative diagnosis [10]. Due to the relapsing/remitting nature of post-COVID symptoms, the following classification has been proposed: Transition Phase (symptoms potentially related to infection; 4–5 weeks), Phase 1 (acute post-COVID symptoms; 5–12 weeks), Phase 2 (symptoms long post-COVID; 12–24 weeks) and Phase 3 (persistent post-COVID symptoms; >24 weeks). Post-acute COVID-19 syndrome (PACS) is considered in patients with persistent post-COVID symptoms (Phase 3) [11]. (Figure 1).

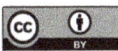

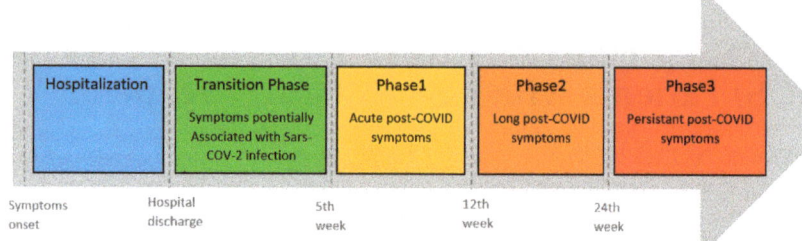

Figure 1. Integrative model of post-COVID symptoms in hospitalized patients showing the Transition Phase (green) and Phases 1 (yellow), 2 (orange) and 3 (red) of post-COVID symptoms [11].

PACS has been described as an expression of a modified aging trajectory induced by SARS-CoV-2 [12]. Aging, defined as the accumulation of unrepaired changes generated in different cells, tissues and organs, depends both on internal and external adaptation mechanisms [13]. At the immunological level, aging is an interaction between the innate immune system, mainly represented by an inflammation cascade [14], and the adaptive immune system, represented by T-lymphocytes [15]. The interaction between inflam-aging and immunosenescence may underlie the pathogenesis of PACS. The accumulation of senescent cells that acquire a secretory phenotype associated with senescence (SASP) [16] has been described, and it is suggested this a phenotypic change is the result of cellular stress secondary to cellular homeostatic mechanisms compromised by SARS-CoV-2. SASP cells release cytokines, chemokines, proteases, reactive metabolites, growth factors, non-coding nucleotides [17], thus effectively activating a chronic inflammatory state.

From hospitalization through to Phase 3, multi-organ signs and symptoms have been reported, including pulmonary [18], cardiovascular [19], metabolic [20], neurocognitive [21], sensory, gastrointestinal [22], psychological [23], dermatological and muscular [11,24]. The pro-inflammatory state associated with COVID-19 and PACS become chronic, [25] provoking cellular senescence [13,16,26]. Muscle weakness, asthenia, sarcopenia, and intolerance to physical exercise [27] in PACS patients is caused by systemic inflammation [28,29], viral infiltration [30], muscle disuse [31], hypoxia [32], malnutrition [33] and adverse drug effects [34].

Further, respiratory fatigue associated with PACS may also be due to respiratory muscle dysfunction, especially the diaphragm [35]. Therefore, it has been suggested that skeletal muscle may be the most affected tissue by the effects of a severe COVID-19 infection. Hence, it is hypothesized that sarcopenia in PACS patients can also affect the masticatory muscles causing fatigue in chewing and possible masticatory distress.

Previous studies have highlighted a link between masticatory dysfunction and sarcopenia. Yoshida et al. reported in 2021 that almost half of the elderly living in Kyoto, Japan has oral hypofunction, defined as a disease not only influenced by aging but also by various factors related to diseases and disorders significantly related to sarcopenia and "frailty" [36]. Kugimiya, Y. et al. in a study of more than 800 elderly (76.5 ± 8.3 years) reported that sarcopenia is observed with a higher frequency in patients diagnosed with oral hypofunction compared to those without; consequently, oral hypofunction appears to be significantly associated with sarcopenia [37].

However, there is currently no evidence in the literature regarding the involvement of the stomatognathic system in PACS patients. We aim to measure the bite force and masticatory performance in PACS patients hospitalized at our center between February 2020 and April 2021.

2. Materials and Methods

We offered a dedicated odontoiatric consultancy to patients diagnosed with PACS attending a dedicated multidisciplinary clinic at Modena University. Patients were selected independently of gravity of PACS and presence of dental signs and symptoms.

Data obtained from medical screening visits of PACS patients included Depression Anxiety Stress Scale (DASS) [38], Body Mass Index (BMI) [39], "dominant hand grip test" (measurement of hand grip strength thanks to a digital dynamometer), "chair stand test" (seconds used for getting up and sitting down 5 times) and "gait speed test" (seconds employed for walking 5 m). The latter two tests are widely used in geriatrics as indicators of motility and frailty among the elderly [40,41].

Asthenia was detected using a predefined checklist of symptoms in which the patient is asked to identify presence and intensity (low, moderate or severe) of muscular symptoms. Sarcopenia was defined according to the European Working Group on Sarcopenia in Older People as low muscle strength, low muscle quantity or quality and low physical performance, adjusted for age and sex [42].

All patients enrolled in the study have PACS symptoms. In our paper, patients are divided into 3 groups: (1) PACS patients with sarcopenia (sarcopenic patients); (2) PACS patients who complain of muscle fatigue but do not fulfill the criteria for diagnosis of sarcopenia (asthenic non-sarcopenic patients); (3) PACS patients without sarcopenia and who do not complain of muscle fatigue (non-asthenic non-sarcopenic patients).

2.1. Short Medical History Interview

Patients were initially subjected to a short medical history associated with COVID-19, including hospitalization, persistence of PACS symptoms, possible presence of temporomandibular disorders and presence of parafunctions.

2.2. Anatomo-Functional Analysis

A palpatory analysis was performed, according to Slavicek [43], to assess the presence of pain in the head and neck muscles and TMJ (Temporo Mandibular Joint) dysfunctions. An extra-oral palpation of the shoulders, neck, atlanto-occipital region, sternocleidomastoid, homohyoid, TMJ in static and opening, posterior joint space, anterior temporal, median and posterior, superficial and digastric masseter was performed.

Intra-oral palpation of deep masseter, medial pterygoid, lateral pterygoid, mylohyoid and tongue was also performed.

The palpation of the TMJ was carried out both at a superficial and intra-articular level to assess the posterior joint space. Any clicks and squeaks heard during jaw opening movements were noted.

The mandibular limit movements of each patient were assessed with the aid of a ruler. Zero was positioned at the incisal edge between 1.1 and 2.1; the mm of maximum opening, right and left lateral movement and protrusion were measured. Maximum opening of >40 mm was considered normal. Laterality assessments were personalized (single patient comparison) according to the movement of the jaw in either direction. Protrusion was measured in mm without any value considered normal. All measurements considered the patients' overjet. Any sagittal axis deviations in the opening and closing route were recorded.

2.3. Intra-Oral Examination

An intra-oral physical examination was performed for each patient. Any missing teeth, prosthetic teeth (crowns on natural teeth or implants, veneers, bridges, pontic elements or teeth in resin belonging to removable partial prosthesis [RPP]), decayed teeth, filled teeth, teeth with non-carious cervical lesion (NCCL), heavily abraded teeth, the level of oral hygiene (excellent, good or poor) and the state of the mucous membranes (presence inflammation, erythematous or hyperplastic areas) were noted. Pockets or pathologies of the periodontium were assessed with periodontal probing. Probing <3.5 mm was considered physiological [44].

2.4. Bite Force Measurement

We measured bite force with the FlexiForce® A201 piezoresistive force transducer (Tekscan, Boston, MA, USA), see Figure 2a. The transducer has a load range up to 440 N, which is suitable for use with adults, and a sensitivity of 0.01 V/N [45]. The force transducer is inserted into a homemade "sandwich structure," consisting of two 8×1 mm discs, made of thermoformed plastic material covered with an aluminum sheet, see Figure 2b. Discs are placed above and below the FlexiForce® force sensor, held in place by a layer of double-sided adhesive tape, according to the manufacturer's recommendation in the FlexiForce® user manual [46]. The function of the plastic disc is to ensure that all lines of force between the upper and lower teeth are conveyed through that area. Because the sensor does not tolerate heat and sterilization [45], the FlexiForce® strip is placed in a disposable plastic shield, used in dentistry for digital intra-oral radiographs. Adequate expression of force is maintained by the maximum thickness of 4 mm, enabling muscle fiber movement at an optimal length [47,48]. Calibration of the sensor was based on data in the literature [45].

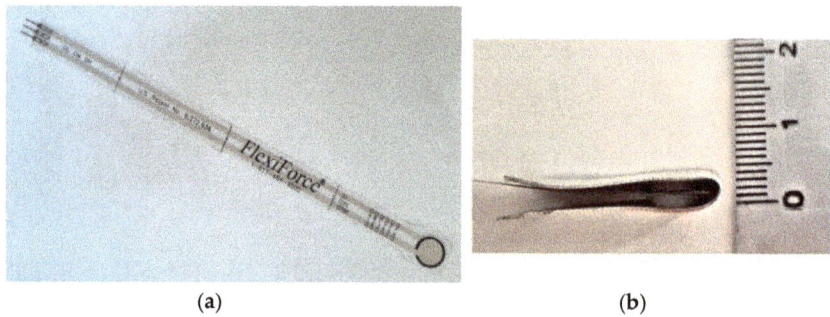

Figure 2. (**a**) FlexiForce® piezoresistive sensor. (**b**) The designed housing with the thermo-molded discs covered with an aluminum sheet.

The two FlexiForce® sensors were connected to an electrical circuit with a voltage of 5 V, powered by a lithium battery. The circuit consists of an "Arduino Uno" controller, to which an LCD screen is connected and displays pressure data. This corresponds to the force expressed in Newtons (N) exerted by the patient during the chewing test (Figure 3).

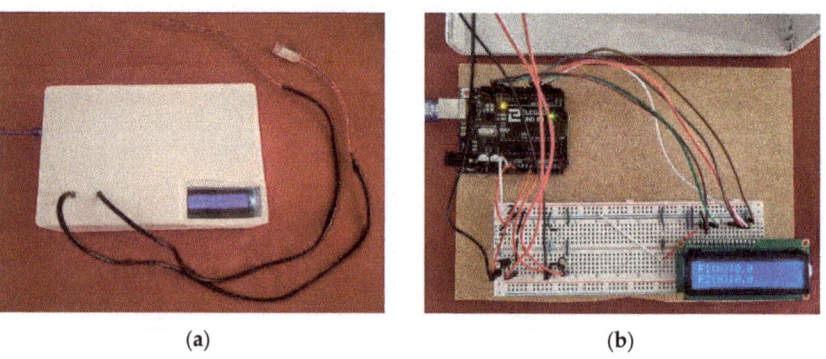

Figure 3. (**a**) External view of the gnathodynamometer with piezoresistive sensors. (**b**) Gnathodynamometer's electronics.

During the design phase of the device, an update frequency of 1.5 Hz for the chewing value was established, and the numerical precision was set to a single decimal digit without approximation. A threshold of 20 N was determined to return a null value [45] and, given the instrumental linear response, measurable and admissible values without losing generality range between 20–320 N.

The sensors were bitten by the patients between the first molars, if present, or between the most posterior teeth. Measurements were taken in the rest position and the maximal chewing force, which was recorded three times.

2.5. Chewing Gum Mixing Ability Test

Garfield® 30 mm long strips of "blue raspberry" (blue) and "all fruits" (red) flavor gum were manually stuck together and used for the chewing gum test. Patients were asked to chew the two strips of gum for 20 mastication cycles [49–51] in a seated upright position. The chewed sample was spat in a plastic bag and temporarily stored in a refrigerator (16 °C).

All gum samples were prepared for analysis by flattening them to a 1 mm thick disk. Then they were photographed from both sides with a Nikon reflex camera (300 dpi resolution) at a standard distance of 10 cm in the same room and with the same lighting conditions [52]. Digitalization of the chewed samples has always been performed within a few hours of the chewing test. Figure 4 shows two examples of chewed gum.

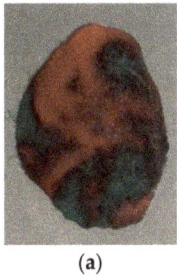 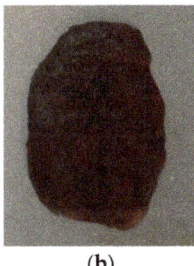

(a)   (b)

Figure 4. (a) chewing gum chewed by a patient with poor chewing efficiency. (b) Chewing gum chewed by a patient with excellent chewing efficiency.

We performed an opto-electrical analysis of the gum photographs to evaluate the degree of color mixing with the ViewGum© software [53] (Figure 5). Variance of hue (VOH), an indication of the logarithmic association with the number of chewing cycles, was used to assess the gum samples; a high VOH indicates poorly mixed colors from poor chewing, and a low VOH indicates well mixed colors from adequate chewing [52]. The results were displayed as "Ch 0 St. Dev" in the ViewGum© software [53].

2.6. Statistical Analysis

Statistical analysis was performed using STATA® software version 17 (StataCorp. 2021. Stata Statistical Software: Release 17. College Station, TX, USA: StataCorp LLC.). The KolmogorovSmirnov test was used to evaluate the normality of the data, and Levene tests were used to assess the homogeneity of variances. We used the parametric tests when assuming the normality of the data distribution and homogeneity of variances. Descriptive statistics were presented for baseline demographic clinical characteristics for the entire group. Continuous variables were presented as mean, standard deviation (SD), minimum (min) and maximum (max) and were compared between subgroups using ANOVA test. A $p < 0.05$ was considered statistically significant.

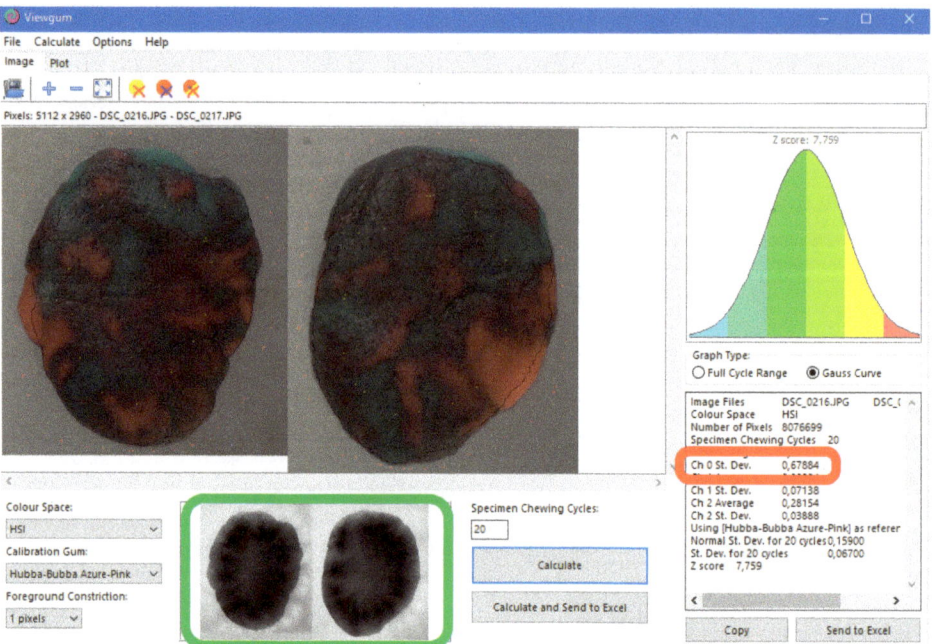

Figure 5. ViewGum© software user interface immediately after loading two images of a chewed gum sample for 20 mastication cycles. The images were obtained by scanning both sides of the flattened gum. The software separates the area of interest from the background as shown by the thumbnail images (green circle). Mouse tracks (yellow and red dots in the main images) can be added or deleted for segmentation. The numerical results are displayed on the right. The VOH value (displayed as "Ch 0 St. Dev" and indicated by an orange box) are calculated; higher VOH correspond to poorer chewing capacity (low color mix).

3. Results

A total of 23 patients out of 35 approached consented to participate in the current study; 12 patients refused. Most were male ($n = 17/23$; 73%), and the mean patient age was 62 ± 7.4 (range 50–75) years old. Patients were hospitalized for COVID-19 infection between February 2020–April 2021. According to PACS muscular symptoms, patients were grouped as sarcopenic ($n = 13/23$; 57%), asthenic non-sarcopenic ($n = 5/23$; 22%) and non-asthenic non-sarcopenic ($n = 5/23$; 22%).

Anxiety (DASS A), depression (DASS D) and stress (DASS S) indices in most patients were within normal ranges [38] (Table 1). Mean patient BMI was 29.5, with value ranges between 41.7 and 21.6. Interestingly, there was no relationship found between BMI and chewing efficacy/efficiency. There was also no relevant difference in BMI between sarcopenic and non-sarcopenic patients. The dominant hand grip test mean values were lower in sarcopenic subjects compared to non-asthenic non-sarcopenic ones (Table 2).

Along with asthenic patients, sarcopenic patients had slower and more strenuous movements, as evidenced in lower gait speed test values compared to non-asthenic non-sarcopenic patients $p = 0.001$, see Figure 6 and Table 2.

Table 1. Intra-oral dental visit and DASS questionnaire results: medium values of missing teeth, crowns, pontic elements or part of Removable Partial Prosthesis (RPP), caries, filled teeth, teeth with Non-Carious Cervical Lesion (NCCL) and Decay Missing Filled Teeth (DMFT); DASS-A; DASS-D; DASS-S.

	Total (n = 23)	Sarcopenic (n = 13, 56.5)	Asthenic Non-Sarcopenic (n = 5, 21.7)	Non Asthenic Non-Sarcopenic (n = 5, 21.7)	p-Value
Missing teeth	5.5 ± 6.8 (0–28)	8.1 ± 7.9 (1–28)	2.0 ± 2.9 (0–7)	2.4 ± 2.7 (0–7)	0.118
Crown	4.3 ± 6.7 (0–28)	4.7 ± 8.1 (0–28)	4.0 ± 6.3 (0–15)	3.6 ± 3.5 (0–9)	0.944
Pontic elements or part of RPP	2.0 ± 4.5 (0–18)	3.0 ± 5.7 (0–18)	1.2 ± 1.7 (0–4)	0.4 ± 0.5 (0–1)	0.507
Teeth present (natural or prosthetic)	25.8 ± 4.8 (13–32)	23.9 ± 5.2 (13–29)	29.6 ± 2.4 (27–32)	27.0 ± 3.1 (22–30)	0.063
Decayed teeth	1.4 ± 1.8 (0–8)	2.0 ± 2.1 (0–8)	0.8 ± 0.8 (0–2)	0.6 ± 0.5 (0–1)	0.235
Filled teeth	2.3 ± 2.6 (0–7)	2.3 ± 2.9 (0–7)	3.0 ± 1.6 (1–5)	2.0 ± 2.8 (0–6)	0.834
Teeth with NCCL	2.9 ± 4.1 (0–14)	1.6 ± 3.8 (0–14)	3.4 ± 3.4 (0–8)	5.8 ± 4.6 (0–11)	0.145
DMFT	12.5 ± 7.1 (3–28)	15.0 ± 7.1 (3–28)	9.8 ± 7.7 (4–23)	8.6 ± 3.7 (3–13)	0.143
DASS-A	4.6 ± 4.4 (0–14)	5.3 ± 5.0 (0–14)	6.0 ± 2.7 (4–9)	1.5 ± 2.3 (0–5)	0.293
DASS-D	4.9 ± 5.1 (0–18)	5.6 ± 5.5 (0–18)	6.3 ± 5.1 (2–12)	2.0 ± 4.0 (0–8)	0.441
DASS-S	6.6 ± 4.7 (0–17)	8.0 ± 4.7 (3–17)	7.7 ± 2.5 (5–10)	2.0 ± 3.4 (0–7)	0.078

Table 2. Comparison of the measurements obtained: DMFT, Value of Hue (VOH), hand grip test, gait speed test, chair stand test and bite force measured in the three groups of patients.

	Total (n = 23)	Sarcopenic (n = 13, 56.5)	Asthenic Non-Sarcopenic (n = 5, 21.7)	Non-Asthenic Non-Sarcopenic (n = 5, 21.7)	p-Value
DMFT	12.5 ± 7.1 (3–28)	15.0 ± 7.1 (3–28)	9.8 ± 7.7 (4–23)	8.6 ± 3.7 (3–13)	0.143
VOH	0.33 ± 0.16 (0.13–0.68)	0.40 ± 0.14 (0.25–0.68)	0.24 ± 0.11 (0.12–0.4)	0.22 ± 0.07 (0.18–0.35)	0.02
Hand grip test	24.2 ± 7.0 (9.2–35.1)	23.4 ± 6.5 (10.1–34.4)	27.6 ± 4.9 (19.2–31.9)	23.1 ± 10.1 (9.2–35.1)	0.501
Gait speed test *	3.6 ± 0.7 (2.6–5.2)	4.1 ± 0.7 (2.9–5.2)	3.2 ± 0.2 (3.0–3.6)	2.8 ± 0.2 (8.5–14.3)	0.001
Chair stand test	12.7 ± 2.7 (8.5–18.7)	13.2 ± 2.9 (9.5–18.7)	13.5 ± 2.2 (10.4–16.3)	10.7 ± 2.3 (8.5–14.3)	0.189
Bite force *	168.5 ± 69.9 (35.5–332.8)	122.4 ± 41.9 (35.5–173.5)	208.5 ± 41.8 (142.3–246.1)	248.2 ± 55.2 (197.5–332.8)	<0.001

* Non-asthenic non-sarcopenic vs. sarcopenic; non-asthenic non-sarcopenic vs. asthenic non-sarcopenic.

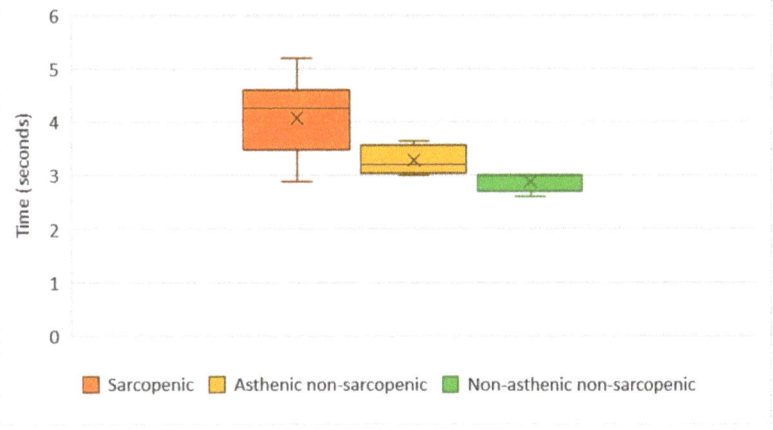

Figure 6. Walking time of the three patient groups: sarcopenic (orange), asthenic non-sarcopenic (yellow) and non-asthenic non-sarcopenic (green).

3.1. Short Medical History Interview

Only 9/23 (39%) were admitted to the Intensive Care Unit (ICU). All ICU admitted patients had post-intensive care syndrome (PICS), reporting general motor difficulties within the first few weeks after discharge [54,55].

Parafunctions were recorded in 8/23 (35%) patients, and one of them reported that nocturnal bruxism began right after discharge, when post-COVID symptoms arose. The reason for the onset cannot be precisely defined, but it can be assumed that it is caused by anxiety and stress—in fact, this patient had very high DASS values. Table 1 reports results about the Depression, Anxiety, and Stress Scale (DASS) questionnaire.

Twenty-three percent of patients reported TMDs (Temporo Mandibular Disorders) before admission, and all of them belong to sarcopenic or asthenic groups. Among the 13 sarcopenic patients, 3 reported spontaneous or chewing pain in the masseter, which appeared shortly after discharge. Two of those offered additional information, specifying motor difficulties associated with the opening and closure of the jaw.

3.2. Anatomo-Functional Analysis

Pain on palpation was recorded according to the muscle location; sternocleidomastoid/occipital/trapexious in 26% (6/23 patients), the mid-anterior temporal in 22% (5/23 patients), mylohyoid in 13% (3/23 patients) and lateral pterygoid in 9% (2/23 patients). No particular areas of muscle tension or inflammation were detected. No patients reported muscle pain during the bite force measurement, so the pain on palpation reported by the subjects is not so severe that it could significantly affect the bite force measurement.

During mandibular movements, noises from the TMJ (Temporo Mandibular Joint) were detected in 11/23 patients (48%), and pain during the jaw opening and closing was recorded in 3/23 (13%). Mandibular opening was normal in 20/23 (87%) patients. Lateral movements were symmetrical, and protrusion was perceivable for most patients; only one patient (sarcopenic) had difficult control of all mandibular movements. There were no differences among the patient groups revealed in terms of any anatomo-functional analysis.

3.3. Intra-Oral Examination

The intra-oral dental examination revealed various critical issues. Oral mucosa showed a normal trophism. Marginal gingivitis was found in 6/23 (26%) patients characterized by the presence of plaque and calculus. Almost half of all patients (n = 11/23; 47.8%) had a poor level of oral hygiene, although periodontal probes were non-physiological in only 4/23 (17%) patients. Table 1 outlines the quantitative measurements from the oral investigations. The overall mean DMFT (Decayed Missing Filled Teeth) was 12.5 ± 7.1. According to study groups, sarcopenic patients displayed a worse overall dental health compared to asthenic non sarcopenic and non-asthenic non-sarcopenic patients.

Comparing the index of each subject, DMFT was higher in sarcopenic patients; no correlation between NCCL and symptoms of sarcopenia or asthenia in PACS patients was found.

3.4. Bite Force Mesurament

According to patient groups, bite force was lowest among sarcopenic patients and highest among the non-asthenic non-sarcopenic patients (Figure 7 and Table 2). In particular, sarcopenic patients have an average decreased bite force of 125.8 N compared to non-asthenic non-sarcopenic subjects and a decreased bite force of 86.1 N compared to asthenic non-sarcopenic subjects. Figure 7 shows the variations in bite force compared to dominant hand force. The difference in bite force among the three groups was much more evident than the hand force. We have registered a maximum bite force value of 332.8 N, while with the hand grip test, the maximum value measured was 47.2 N.

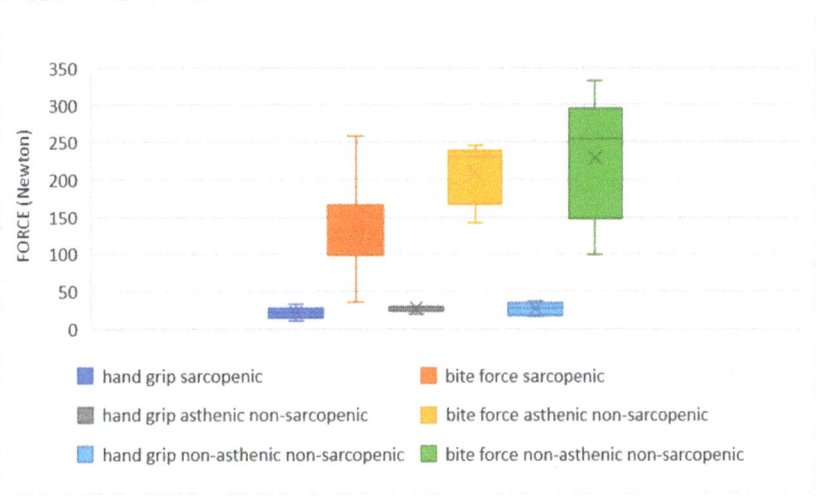

Figure 7. Comparison between hand-grip force and bite force for the three groups of patients.

3.5. Chewing Gum Mixing Ability Test

The VOH ranged between 0.127 and 0.678. The highest values (inefficient chewing) were observed in sarcopenic patients, compared to non-asthenic non-sarcopenic and asthenic non-sarcopenic subjects (Figure 8 and Table 2). Sarcopenic patients showed an average VOH of 0.403; non-asthenic non-sarcopenic patients showed an average VOH value of 0.22. This difference is statistically significant.

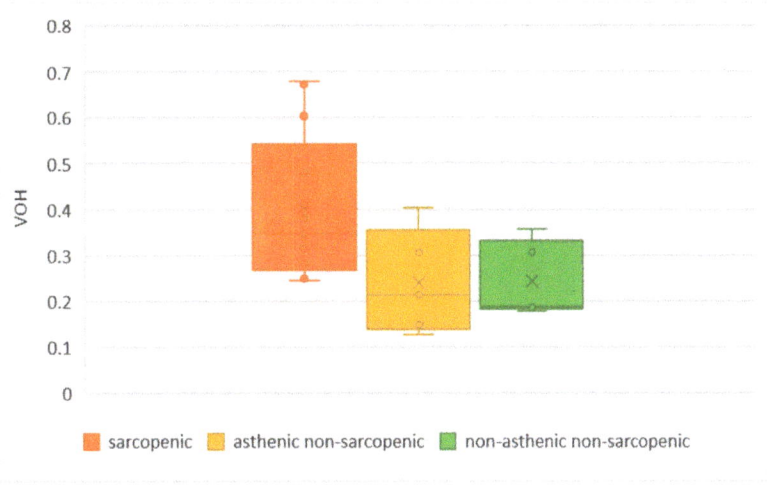

Figure 8. Chewing efficiency: comparison of VOH values between sarcopenic, asthenic non-sarcopenic and non-asthenic non-sarcopenic subjects.

We also compared the VOH with the DMFT and the number of teeth in the arch (prosthetic or natural). Figures 9 and 10 demonstrate how oral health, especially of the teeth, was correlated with patients' masticatory performance.

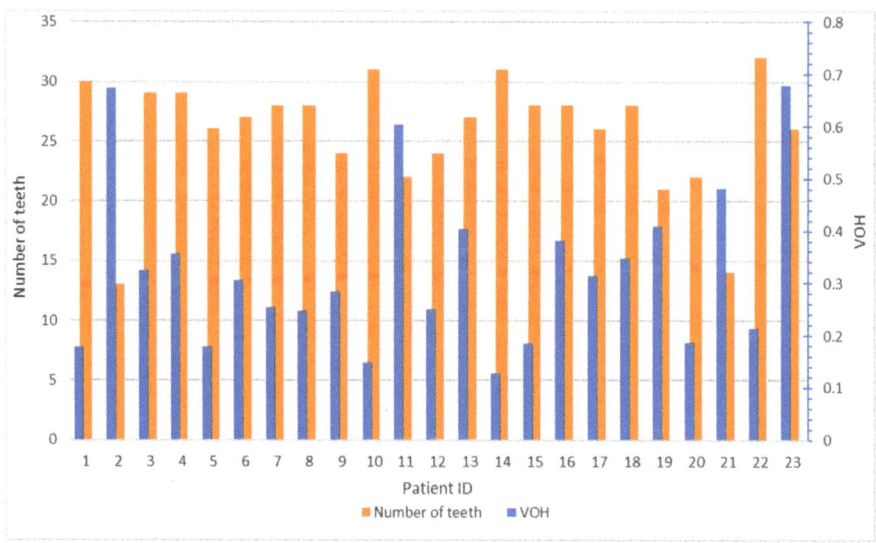

Figure 9. Comparison between VOH (in blue) and the number of prosthetic/natural teeth present in the arches (in orange). As can be seen from the graph, patients with fewer teeth tend to have a higher VOH score.

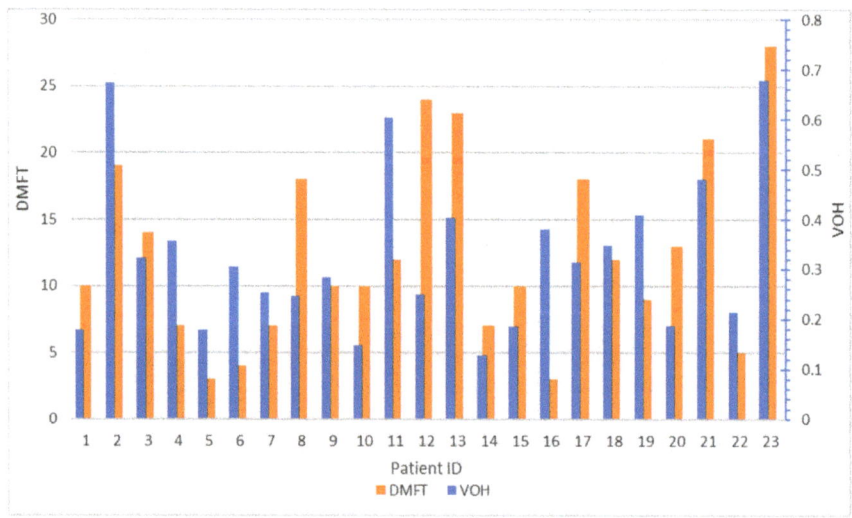

Figure 10. Comparison between VOH (in blue) and DMFT (in orange). From the figure, it is possible to appreciate how the higher the DMFT index, the higher the VOH.

4. Discussion

This research includes both intra-oral and extra-oral physical examination. This choice is motivated by the need to observe a variety of possible effects of PACS or COVID-19 in the areas of dental interest (teeth, mucous membranes and periodontium).

4.1. Short Medical History Interview

Stress, anxiety and emotional factors can create parafunctional problems, such as nocturnal grinding or locking, or exacerbate those already present [56,57], and it is important to consider psychological factors when investigating dysfunctional problems.

The severity of COVID-19 affects the symptoms and incidence of PACS [12]. With the anamnestic interview, the patients who were admitted to intensive care unit reported the difficulties encountered after discharge. It is, therefore, evident that post-intensive care syndrome (PISC) can affect the stomatognathic system and can also leave chewing problems.

4.2. Anatomo-Functional Analysis

Some patients responded positively to muscle palpation, indicating specific areas of pain. In many of them, dysfunctional signs and symptoms were found, often mild. In general, it can be said that the TMJ does not perform its function perfectly in all subjects. It is not known exactly the reason behind the slight dysfunctions highlighted in these PACS subjects because there is no data of the anatomo-functional analysis before the COVID-19 infection. It can be hypothesized that the pain in the cervico-facial muscles found post-COVID may be part of the musculoskeletal symptoms characteristic of PACS; nevertheless, further studies are needed to confirm this hypothesis.

4.3. Intra-Oral Examination

The surveys did not reveal periodontal problems in most patients. The only non-physiological probes (>3 mm) were observed in those patients with a poor level of oral hygiene and were attributable to gingival inflammation due to tartar and plaque. No cases of obvious inflammatory gingival problems have been found, so it can be said that the systemic inflammation underlying PACS does not affect oral soft tissues.

Third molars were not taken into consideration, thus reducing the maximum DMFT value to 28. The mean DMFT was 12.5 ± 7.1, hence the oral health status of the PACS subjects under examination is worse than the values found in the literature [58]. The reason may be that the PACS patient shifted attention to more important health problems—even hospitalization did not help to maintain proper oral hygiene. Many of these patients had to wear an oxygen insufflation mask for some time and were intubated [59]. Most patients reported that they did not go to the dentist prior to the COVID-19 infection.

The NCCL results are in line with a 2020 meta-analysis [60]. Many studies were not able to confirm a positive association between occlusal loading and abfraction. The literature suggests that dentin demineralization promotes NCCL formation from an early stage, while occlusal stress is an etiological factor contributing to the progression of these lesions [61].

4.4. Bite Force Measurement

The FlexiForce® device has already been used in the related literature [62,63]. When inserting a device between the first or second molar, the mouth opens no more than 2–3 mm interincisal distance. This means that the condyles remain almost centered in the temporal fossa, i.e., in a centric position.

During the measurement, it was difficult to ensure that the sensor remained correctly interposed between the cusps of the teeth. The occlusal table is not as flat as the sensor turns out to be. The thermoplastic material of the discs, which is elastic, helps to overcome this problem. The aluminum sheet allows the correct positioning of the cusps with respect to the sensor, but it can also represent a disadvantage; if during the first detection the thermo-molded disc is moved outside the sensitive area of the Flexi-Force®, the subsequent measurements are invalid. To address this problem, when the aluminum housing undergoes a clear plastic deformation, it is replaced.

The measurement takes place simultaneously on the right and left side, thus allowing one to quantify any masticatory asymmetries. However, for the purposes of the study, the average value of bite force between the right and the left was considered of most interest.

4.5. Chewing Gum Mixing Ability Test

The most important predictors of chewing efficiency are the number of pairs of occluding teeth, the bite force, the flow of saliva, prosthetic reconstructions, the strength and coordination of the tongue and cheeks, as well as age and sex [64,65]. Cognitive status and intra-oral sensitivity are also associated with chewing function [52]. This study only considers age, number of teeth and bite force.

The two-color chewing gum test is documented as a simple and effective test that can be used in the clinical setting [66]. The literature recommends the chewing gum mixing test to evaluate interindividual differences in chewing efficiency in clinical and research settings, in both prosthetic and non-prosthetic patients [67]. The simplicity of the optoelectronic assessment could help establish widespread screening for masticatory deficiencies. Furthermore, application in geriatrics or special care could help visualize oral-functionality or dental comorbidities.

From the data obtained through Viewgum©, it is evident that sarcopenic patients have a lower degree of masticatory performance than those without muscle symptoms (non-asthenic non-sarcopenic patients). This may be due to both decreased muscle function, caused by PACS, but also an increased DMFT. Comparisons of the VOH against the DMFT (Figure 10) or the number of teeth (Figure 9) highlight that chewing efficiency depends on the state of the oral health. Since it can be difficult to increase the muscular performance of sarcopenic PACS patients, it is advisable to improve the state of oral health and to rehabilitate missing teeth.

4.6. Limits of the Study

The lack of data on the chewing performance of patients before COVID-19 infection and the small number of subjects prevent proving that PACS was the actual cause of the decreased chewing performance. Moreover, this study does not allow us to detect improvement or deterioration in muscle performance over time.

We do not have the possibility to do an X-ray examination. For this reason, we only conducted an intra-oral examination that does not allow us to collect data about interproximal caries, periapical lesions and root fractures.

In this study, we used Garfield® chewing gums. We remark that these chewing gums are not the same used and validated in the previous studies. Validated chewing gums (either Hubba Bubba® or HueCheck®) were not readily available in our country at the moment of the investigation. We selected Garfield® chewing gums because they are the most similar to Hubba Bubba®.

We remark that bite force is different from masticatory force because the clenching movement of the mouth is different from the chewing movement. For this reason, the study cannot affirm the correlation between PACS and masticatory force.

5. Conclusions

In conclusion, the study showed that PACS people with sarcopenia have an average bite force of 122.4 Newton (N). This value is 86.1 N lower than asthenic non-sarcopenic patients (average bite force of 208.5 N) and 125.8 N lower than non-asthenic non-sarcopenic patients (average bite force of 248.2 N), As regards chewing efficiency, sarcopenic patients showed an average VOH increase of 0.18 compared to non-asthenic non-sarcopenic ones. Patients who complained only of asthenia (asthenic non-sarcopenic) were found to have lower values of bite force and masticatory efficacy than those who did not have muscular symptoms (non-asthenic non-sarcopenic) but higher values than those who suffered from sarcopenia (sarcopenic).

The piezoresistive sensor gnathodynamometer proved to be a valid bite force measurement tool. This tool can be a good alternative to other motor tests used to evaluate muscle effectiveness (such as the dominant hand grip test). Further studies on larger groups of subjects will be needed to validate their clinical use.

Oral health in most PACS patients appears to be compromised; it is, therefore, advisable to direct these patients towards a multi-disciplinary-rehabilitation path, addressing dental issues as well as all functional problems already present or occurring in the post-hospitalization.

Author Contributions: Conceptualization, B.D.P. and G.G. (Giovanni Guaraldi); methodology, G.G. (Giovanni Guaraldi), B.D.P.; software, R.K.K.; validation, L.B. and P.B.; formal analysis, R.K.K. and L.B.; investigation, L.B. and B.D.P.; resources, G.G. (Giovanni Guaraldi) and R.K.K.; writing—original draft preparation, L.B. and G.G. (Giovanna Garuti); writing—review and editing, L.B. and G.G. (Giovanna Garuti); supervision, U.C., P.B. and G.G. (Giovanna Garuti); project administration, U.C. and P.B. All authors have read and agreed to the published version of the manuscript.

Funding: This research received no external funding.

Institutional Review Board Statement: All subjects gave informed consent for inclusion before participating in the study. This study was conducted in accordance with the Declaration of Helsinki, and the protocol was approved by the ethic committee of "Area Vasta Emilia Nord" with the project identification code number 396/2020.

Informed Consent Statement: Informed consent was obtained from all subjects involved in the study.

Data Availability Statement: Not applicable.

Conflicts of Interest: The authors declare no conflict of interest.

References

1. Imai, K.; Tanaka, H. SARS-CoV-2 Infection and Significance of Oral Health Management in the Era of "the New Normal with COVID-19". *Int. J. Mol. Sci.* **2021**, *22*, 6527. [CrossRef]
2. Huang, N.; Pérez, P.; Kato, T.; Mikami, Y.; Okuda, K.; Gilmore, R.C.; Conde, C.D.; Gasmi, B.; Stein, S.; Beach, M.; et al. SARS-CoV-2 infection of the oral cavity and saliva. *Nat. Med.* **2021**, *27*, 892–903. [CrossRef] [PubMed]
3. Mulchandani, R.; Lyngdoh, T.; Kakkar, A.K. Deciphering the COVID-19 cytokine storm: Systematic review and meta-analysis. *Eur. J. Clin. Investig.* **2021**, *51*, e13429. [CrossRef] [PubMed]
4. Sakaguchi, W.; Kubota, N.; Shimizu, T.; Saruta, J.; Fuchida, S.; Kawata, A.; Yamamoto, Y.; Sugimoto, M.; Yakeishi, M.; Tsukinoki, K. Existence of SARS-CoV-2 Entry Molecules in the Oral Cavity. *Int. J. Mol. Sci.* **2020**, *21*, 6000. [CrossRef] [PubMed]
5. Xu, H.; Zhong, L.; Deng, J.; Peng, J.; Dan, H.; Zeng, X.; Li, T.; Chen, Q. High expression of ACE2 receptor of 2019-nCoV on the epithelial cells of oral mucosa. *Int. J. Oral Sci.* **2020**, *12*, 8. [CrossRef] [PubMed]
6. Mason, R.J. Pathogenesis of COVID-19 from a cell biology perspective. *Eur. Respir. J.* **2020**, *55*, 2000607. [CrossRef] [PubMed]
7. Gu, S.X.; Tyagi, T.; Jain, K.; Gu, V.W.; Lee, S.H.; Hwa, J.M.; Kwan, J.M.; Krause, D.S.; Lee, A.I.; Halene, S.; et al. Thrombocytopathy and endotheliopathy: Crucial contributors to COVID-19 thromboinflammation. *Nat. Rev. Cardiol.* **2020**, *18*, 194–209. [CrossRef]
8. Fabrizi, F.; Alfieri, C.M.; Cerutti, R.; Lunghi, G.; Messa, P. COVID-19 and Acute Kidney Injury: A Systematic Review and Meta-Analysis. *Pathogens* **2020**, *9*, 1052. [CrossRef]
9. Sultan, S.; Altayar, O.; Siddique, S.M.; Davitkov, P.; Feuerstein, J.D.; Lim, J.K.; Falck-Ytter, Y.; El-Serag, H.B. AGA Institute Rapid Review of the Gastrointestinal and Liver Manifestations of COVID-19, Meta-Analysis of International Data, and Recommendations for the Consultative Management of Patients with COVID-19. *Gastroenterology* **2020**, *159*, 320–334.e27. [CrossRef]
10. Herridge, M.S.; Tansey, C.; Matté, A.; Tomlinson, G.; Diaz-Granados, N.; Cooper, A.; Guest, C.; Mazer, D.; Mehta, S.; Stewart, T.; et al. Functional Disability 5 Years after Acute Respiratory Distress Syndrome. *N. Engl. J. Med.* **2011**, *364*, 1293–1304. [CrossRef]
11. Fernández-De-Las-Peñas, C.; Palacios-Ceña, D.; Gómez-Mayordomo, V.; Cuadrado, M.L.; Florencio, L.L. Defining Post-COVID Symptoms (Post-Acute COVID, Long COVID, Persistent Post-COVID): An Integrative Classification. *Int. J. Environ. Res. Public Health* **2021**, *18*, 2621. [CrossRef]
12. Taquet, M.; Dercon, Q.; Luciano, S.; Geddes, J.R.; Husain, M.; Harrison, P.J. Incidence, co-occurrence, and evolution of long-COVID features: A 6-month retrospective cohort study of 273,618 survivors of COVID-19. *PLoS Med.* **2021**, *18*, e1003773. [CrossRef] [PubMed]
13. Cohen, A.A. Complex systems dynamics in aging: New evidence, continuing questions. *Biogerontology* **2016**, *17*, 205–220. [CrossRef] [PubMed]
14. 2021 Alzheimer's Disease Facts and Figures. Available online: https://alz-journals.onlinelibrary.wiley.com/doi/10.1002/alz.12328#:~{}:text=An%20estimated%206.2%20million%20Americans,prevent%2C%20slow%20or%20cure%20AD (accessed on 17 December 2022).
15. COVID-19 Associated with Long-Term Cognitive Dysfunction, Acceleration of Alzheimer's Symptoms. Available online: https://aaic.alz.org/releases_2021/covid-19-cognitive-impact.asp (accessed on 19 January 2023).

16. Fulop, T.; Larbi, A.; Dupuis, G.; Le Page, A.; Frost, E.H.; Cohen, A.A.; Witkowski, J.M.; Franceschi, C. Immunosenescence and Inflamm-Aging as Two Sides of the Same Coin: Friends or Foes? *Front. Immunol.* **2018**, *8*, 1960. [CrossRef] [PubMed]
17. Coppé, J.-P.; Patil, C.K.; Rodier, F.; Sun, Y.; Muñoz, D.P.; Goldstein, J.; Nelson, P.S.; Desprez, P.-Y.; Campisi, J. Senescence-Associated Secretory Phenotypes Reveal Cell-Nonautonomous Functions of Oncogenic RAS and the p53 Tumor Suppressor. *PLoS Biol.* **2008**, *6*, e301. [CrossRef]
18. Salehi, S.; Reddy, S.; Gholamrezanezhad, A. Long-term Pulmonary Consequences of Coronavirus Disease 2019 (COVID-19): What we know and what to expect. *J. Thorac. Imaging* **2020**, *35*, W87–W89. [CrossRef]
19. Puntmann, V.O.; Carerj, M.L.; Wieters, I.; Fahim, M.; Arendt, C.; Hoffmann, J.; Shchendrygina, A.; Escher, F.; Vasa-Nicotera, M.; Zeiher, A.M.; et al. Outcomes of Cardiovascular Magnetic Resonance Imaging in Patients Recently Recovered from Coronavirus Disease 2019 (COVID-19). *JAMA Cardiol.* **2020**, *5*, 1265–1273. [CrossRef]
20. Sathish, T.; Anton, M.C.; Sivakumar, T. New-onset diabetes in 'long COVID'. *J. Diabetes* **2021**, *13*, 693–694. [CrossRef]
21. Wang, F.; Kream, R.M.; Stefano, G.B. Long-term respiratory and neurological sequelae of COVID-19. *Med. Sci. Monit.* **2020**, *26*, e928996. [CrossRef]
22. Phipps, M.M.; Barraza, L.H.; Lasota, E.D.; Sobieszczyk, M.E.; Pereira, M.R.; Zheng, E.X.; Fox, A.N.; Zucker, J.; Verna, E.C. Acute Liver Injury in COVID-19: Prevalence and Association with Clinical Outcomes in a Large U.S. Cohort. *Hepatology* **2020**, *72*, 807–817. [CrossRef]
23. Troyer, E.A.; Kohn, J.N.; Hong, S. Are we facing a crashing wave of neuropsychiatric sequelae of COVID-19? Neuropsychiatric symptoms and potential immunologic mechanisms. *Brain. Behav. Immun.* **2020**, *87*, 34–39. [CrossRef]
24. Karaarslan, F.; Demircioğlu Güneri, F.; Kardeş, S. Postdischarge rheumatic and musculoskeletal symptoms following hospitalization for COVID-19: Prospective follow-up by phone interviews. *Rheumatol. Int.* **2021**, *41*, 1263–1271. [CrossRef]
25. Bektas, A.; Schurman, S.H.; Franceschi, C.; Ferrucci, L. A public health perspective of aging: Do hyper-inflammatory syndromes such as COVID-19, SARS, ARDS, cytokine storm syndrome, and post-ICU syndrome accelerate short- and long-term inflammaging? *Immun. Ageing* **2020**, *17*, 23. [CrossRef]
26. Delgado-Alonso, C.; Valles-Salgado, M.; Delgado-Álvarez, A.; Yus, M.; Gómez-Ruiz, N.; Jorquera, M.; Polidura, C.; Gil, M.J.; Marcos, A.; Matías-Guiu, J.; et al. Cognitive dysfunction associated with COVID-19: A comprehensive neuropsychological study. *J. Psychiatr. Res.* **2022**, *150*, 40–46. [CrossRef] [PubMed]
27. van den Borst, B.; Peters, J.B.; Brink, M.; Schoon, Y.; Bleeker-Rovers, C.P.; Schers, H.; van Hees, H.W.H.; van Helvoort, H.; van den Boogaard, M.; van der Hoeven, H.; et al. Comprehensive Health Assessment 3 Months After Recovery from Acute Coronavirus Disease 2019 (COVID-19). *Clin. Infect. Dis.* **2021**, *73*, e1089. [CrossRef] [PubMed]
28. Bloch, S.; Polkey, M.I.; Griffiths, M.; Kemp, P. Molecular mechanisms of intensive care unit-acquired weakness. *Eur. Respir. J.* **2012**, *39*, 1000–1011. [CrossRef]
29. Wåhlin-Larsson, B.; Wilkinson, D.J.; Strandberg, E.; Hosford-Donovan, A.; Atherton, P.J.; Kadi, F. Mechanistic Links Underlying the Impact of C-Reactive Protein on Muscle Mass in Elderly. *Cell. Physiol. Biochem.* **2017**, *44*, 267–278. [CrossRef] [PubMed]
30. Aschman, T.; Schneider, J.; Greuel, S.; Meinhardt, J.; Streit, S.; Goebel, H.-H.; Büttnerova, I.; Elezkurtaj, S.; Scheibe, F.; Radke, J.; et al. Association Between SARS-CoV-2 Infection and Immune-Mediated Myopathy in Patients Who Have Died. *JAMA Neurol.* **2021**, *78*, 948–960. [CrossRef]
31. de Andrade-Junior, M.C.; de Salles, I.C.D.; de Brito, C.M.M.; Pastore-Junior, L.; Righetti, R.F.; Yamaguti, W.P. Skeletal Muscle Wasting and Function Impairment in Intensive Care Patients with Severe COVID-19. *Front. Physiol.* **2021**, *12*, 640973. [CrossRef]
32. McKenna, H.T.; Murray, A.J.; Martin, D.S. Human adaptation to hypoxia in critical illness. *J. Appl. Physiol.* **2020**, *129*, 656–663. [CrossRef]
33. Wierdsma, N.J.; Kruizenga, H.M.; Konings, L.A.; Krebbers, D.; Jorissen, J.R.; Joosten, M.-H.I.; van Aken, L.H.; Tan, F.M.; van Bodegraven, A.A.; Soeters, M.R.; et al. Poor nutritional status, risk of sarcopenia and nutrition related complaints are prevalent in COVID-19 patients during and after hospital admission. *Clin. Nutr. Espen.* **2021**, *43*, 369. [CrossRef] [PubMed]
34. Soares, M.N.; Eggelbusch, M.; Naddaf, E.; Gerrits, K.H.L.; van der Schaaf, M.; van den Borst, B.; Wiersinga, W.J.; van Vugt, M.; Weijs, P.J.M.; Murray, A.J.; et al. Skeletal muscle alterations in patients with acute COVID-19 and post-acute sequelae of COVID-19. *J. Cachexia Sarcopenia Muscle* **2022**, *13*, 11–22. [CrossRef] [PubMed]
35. Shepherd, S.; Batra, A.; Lerner, D.P. Review of Critical Illness Myopathy and Neuropathy. *Neurohospitalist* **2017**, *7*, 41–48. [CrossRef]
36. Yoshida, M.; Hiraoka, A.; Takeda, C.; Mori, T.; Maruyama, M.; Yoshikawa, M.; Tsuga, K. Oral hypofunction and its relation to frailty and sarcopenia in community-dwelling older people. *Gerodontology* **2022**, *39*, 26–32. [CrossRef] [PubMed]
37. Kugimiya, Y.; Iwasaki, M.; Ohara, Y.; Motokawa, K.; Edahiro, A.; Shirobe, M.; Watanabe, Y.; Obuchi, S.; Kawai, H.; Fujiwara, Y.; et al. Relationship between Oral Hypofunction and Sarcopenia in Community-Dwelling Older Adults: The Otassha Study. *Int. J. Environ. Res. Public Health* **2021**, *18*, 6666. [CrossRef]
38. Višnjić, A.; Veličković, V.; Sokolović, D.; Stanković, M.; Mijatović, K.; Milošević, Z.; Radulović, O. Relationship between the manner of mobile phone use and depression, anxiety, and stress in university students. *Int. J. Environ. Res. Public Health* **2018**, *15*, 697. [CrossRef]
39. Calcolo Indice Massa Corporea—IMC (BMI—Body Mass Index). Available online: https://www.salute.gov.it/portale/nutrizione/dettaglioIMCNutrizione.jsp?lingua=italiano&id=5479&area=nutrizione&menu=vuoto (accessed on 17 December 2022).

40. Fried, L.P.; Tangen, C.M.; Walston, J.; Newman, A.B.; Hirsch, C.; Gottdiener, J.; Seeman, T.; Tracy, R.; Kop, W.J.; Burke, G.; et al. Frailty in Older AdultsEvidence for a Phenotype. *J. Gerontol. Ser. A* **2001**, *56*, M146–M157. [CrossRef]
41. Giornale di Cardiologia. Available online: https://www.giornaledicardiologia.it/archivio/1261/articoli/13935/#:~{}:text=Inparticolare%2Cunavelocita%3E1.0,instabilieridottaautonomia24 (accessed on 17 December 2022).
42. Cruz-Jentoft, A.J.; Bahat, G.; Bauer, J.; Boirie, Y.; Bruyère, O.; Cederholm, T.; Cooper, C.; Landi, F.; Rolland, Y.; Aihie Sayer, A.; et al. Sarcopenia: Revised European consensus on definition and diagnosis. *Age Ageing* **2019**, *48*, 16–31. [CrossRef]
43. Sondaggio Parodontale. Available online: https://www.gengive.org/glossario/sondaggio-parodontale/ (accessed on 17 December 2022).
44. Testa, M.; Di Marco, A.; Pertusio, R.; Van Roy, P.; Cattrysse, E.; Roatta, S. A validation study of a new instrument for low cost bite force measurement. *J. Electromyogr. Kinesiol.* **2016**, *30*, 243–248. [CrossRef]
45. FlexiForce User Manual | Tekscan. Available online: https://www.tekscan.com/support/faqs/flexiforce-user-manual (accessed on 16 May 2022).
46. Manns, A.; Miralles, R.; Palazzi, C. EMG, bite force, and elongation of the masseter muscle under isometric voluntary contractions and variations of vertical dimension. *J. Prosthet. Dent.* **1979**, *42*, 674–682. [CrossRef]
47. Âudio, C.; Fernandes, P.; Glantz, J.; Svensson, S.A.; Bergmark, A. A Novel Sensor for Bite Force Determinations. Available online: http://www.elsevier.com/locate/dental (accessed on 17 December 2022).
48. Anastassiadou, V.; Heath, M.R.; Bartholomew, S. The development of a simple objective test of mastication suitable for older people, using chewing gums. *Gerodontology* **2001**, *18*, 79–86. [CrossRef]
49. Prinz, J.F. Quantitative evaluation of the effect of bolus size and number of chewing strokes on the intra-oral mixing of a two-colour chewing gum. *J. Oral Rehabil.* **1999**, *26*, 243–247. [CrossRef] [PubMed]
50. Schimmel, M.; Leemann, B.; Herrmann, F.R.; Kiliaridis, S.; Schnider, A.; Müller, F. Masticatory function and bite force in stroke patients. *J. Dent. Res.* **2011**, *90*, 230–234. [CrossRef]
51. Buser, R.; Ziltener, V.; Samietz, S.; Fontolliet, M.; Nef, T.; Schimmel, M. Validation of a purpose-built chewing gum and smartphone application to evaluate chewing efficiency. *J. Oral Rehabil.* **2018**, *45*, 845–853. [CrossRef] [PubMed]
52. Fankhauser, N.; Kalberer, N.; Müller, F.; Leles, C.R.; Schimmel, M.; Srinivasan, M. Comparison of smartphone-camera and conventional flatbed scanner images for analytical evaluation of chewing function. *J. Oral Rehabil.* **2020**, *47*, 1496–1502. [CrossRef]
53. ViewGum. Available online: http://www.dhal.com/viewgum.html (accessed on 17 December 2022).
54. Chippa, V.; Aleem, A.; Anjum, F. Post Acute Coronavirus (COVID-19) Syndrome. *StatPearls*. **2022**. Available online: https://www.ncbi.nlm.nih.gov/books/NBK570608/ (accessed on 17 December 2022).
55. PICS. Available online: https://postintensiva.it/la-pics-post-intensive-care-syndrome/ (accessed on 17 December 2022).
56. Kuhn, M.; Türp, J.C.; Türp, J.C.; Myoarthropathien, M.A.A. Risk factors for bruxism. *SWISS Dent. J. SSO* **2018**, *128*, 118–124.
57. Ohrbach, R.; Michelotti, A. The Role of Stress in the Etiology of Oral Parafunction and Myofascial Pain. *Oral Maxillofac. Surg. Clin. N. Am.* **2018**, *30*, 369–379. [CrossRef]
58. Kit, A.; Tamrakar, M.; Jiang, C.M.; Man Lo, E.C.; Man Leung, K.C.; Chu, C.H. A Systematic Review on Caries Status of Older Adults. *Int. J. Environ. Res. Public Health* **2021**, *18*, 10662. [CrossRef]
59. Mańka-Malara, K.; Gawlak, D.; Hovhannisyan, A.; Klikowska, M.; Kostrzewa-Janicka, J. Dental trauma prevention during endotracheal intubation—Review of literature. *Anaesthesiol. Intensive Ther.* **2015**, *47*, 425–429. [CrossRef]
60. Teixeira, D.N.R.; Thomas, R.Z.; Soares, P.V.; Cune, M.S.; Gresnigt, M.M.M.; Slot, D.E. Prevalence of noncarious cervical lesions among adults: A systematic review. *J. Dent.* **2020**, *95*, 103285. [CrossRef]
61. Nascimento, M.M.; Dilbone, D.A.; Pereira, P.N.; Duarte, R.; Geraldeli, S.; Delgado, A.J. Clinical, Cosmetic and Investigational Dentistry Abfraction lesions: Etiology, diagnosis, and treatment options. *Clin. Cosmet. Investig. Dent.* **2016**, *8*, 79–87. [CrossRef] [PubMed]
62. Testa, M.; Rolando, M. Control of jaw-clenching forces in dentate subjects. *J. Orofac. Pain* **2011**, *25*, 250–260. [PubMed]
63. Testa, M.; Geri, T.; Signori, A.; Roatta, S. Visual Feedback of Bilateral Bite Force to Assess Motor Control of the Mandible in Isometric Condition. *Mot. Control.* **2015**, *19*, 312–324. [CrossRef]
64. Ikebe, K.; Matsuda, K.-I.; Kagawa, R.; Enoki, K.; Yoshida, M.; Maeda, Y.; Nokubi, T. Association of masticatory performance with age, gender, number of teeth, occlusal force and salivary flow in Japanese older adults: Is ageing a risk factor for masticatory dysfunction? *Arch. Oral Biol.* **2011**, *56*, 991–996. [CrossRef]
65. Yamada, A.; Kanazawa, M.; Komagamine, Y.; Minakuchi, S. Association between tongue and lip functions and masticatory performance in young dentate adults. *J. Oral Rehabil.* **2015**, *42*, 833–839. [CrossRef] [PubMed]
66. Schimmel, M.; Christou, P.; Miyazaki, H.; Halazonetis, D.; Herrmann, F.R.; Müller, F. A novel colourimetric technique to assess chewing function using two-coloured specimens: Validation and application. *J. Dent.* **2015**, *43*, 955–964. [CrossRef] [PubMed]
67. Silva, L.C.; Nogueira, T.E.; Rios, L.F.; Schimmel, M.; Leles, C.R. Reliability of a two-colour chewing gum test to assess masticatory performance in complete denture wearers. *J. Oral Rehabil.* **2018**, *45*, 301–307. [CrossRef]

Disclaimer/Publisher's Note: The statements, opinions and data contained in all publications are solely those of the individual author(s) and contributor(s) and not of MDPI and/or the editor(s). MDPI and/or the editor(s) disclaim responsibility for any injury to people or property resulting from any ideas, methods, instructions or products referred to in the content.

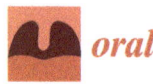

Communication

Oral Toxicities in Cancer Patients, Who Receive Immunotherapy: A Case Series of 24 Patients

Ourania Nicolatou-Galitis [1,*], Amanda Psyrri [2], Nikolaos Tsoukalas [3], Evangelos Galitis [4], Helena Linardou [5], Dimitra Galiti [6], Ilias Athansiadis [7], Despoina Kalapanida [8], Evangelia Razis [8], Nikolaos Katirtzoglou [9], Nikolaos Kentepozidis [10], Paraskevas Kosmidis [11], Flora Stavridi [12], Efthimios Kyrodimos [13], Danai Daliani [9], George Tsironis [14], Giannis Mountzios [15], Sofia Karageorgopoulou [16], Panagiotis Gouveris [17] and Konstantinos Syrigos [18]

1. CureCancer PC, Anastaseos 23, 15561 Athens, Greece
2. B′ Propaideytiki Pathology Clinic, Peripheral General Hospital of Athens, Oncology Department, "Attikon" School of Medicine, National and Kapodistrian University of Athens, 12461 Athens, Greece
3. Oncology Department, 401 General Military Hospital, 11525 Athens, Greece
4. Clinic of Oral Surgery, School of Dentistry, National and Kapodistrian University of Athens, 11527 Athens, Greece
5. 4th Oncology Dept & Comprehensive Clinical Trials Center, Metropolitan Hospital, 18547 Athens, Greece
6. Clinic of Oral Diagnosis and Radiology, School of Dentistry, National and Kapodistrian University of Athens, 11527 Athens, Greece
7. Oncology Clinic, Mitera Hospital, 15123 Athens, Greece
8. 3rd Pathology Oncology Clinic, Hygeia Hospital, 15123 Athens, Greece
9. 1st Medical Oncology Department, Euroclinic of Athens, 11521 Athens, Greece
10. Medical Oncology Clinic, 251 Hellenic Air Force General Hospital, 11527 Athens, Greece
11. 2nd Pathology Oncology Clinic, Hygeia Hospital, 15123 Athens, Greece
12. 4th Pathology Oncology Clinic, Hygeia Hospital, 15123 Athens, Greece
13. ENT Clinic, Hippokration Hospital, School of Medicine, National and Kapodistrian University of Athens, 11527 Athens, Greece
14. Bank of Cyprus Oncology Center, 2006 Nicosia, Cyprus
15. Clinical Trials Unit, 2nd Oncology Department, Henry Dunant Hospital Center, 11526 Athens, Greece
16. IASO Clinic, 3rd Medical Oncology Department, 15123 Athens, Greece
17. 2nd Oncology Clinic, Agios Savvas Hospital, 10447 Athens, Greece
18. 3rd Pathology Clinic, General Hospital for Thoracic Diseases of Athens "Sotiria", School of Medicine, National and Kapodistrian University of Athens, 11527 Athens, Greece
* Correspondence: nicolatou.galitis@hotmail.com; Tel.: +30-6944601529

Citation: Nicolatou-Galitis, O.; Psyrri, A.; Tsoukalas, N.; Galitis, E.; Linardou, H.; Galiti, D.; Athansiadis, I.; Kalapanida, D.; Razis, E.; Katirtzoglou, N.; et al. Oral Toxicities in Cancer Patients, Who Receive Immunotherapy: A Case Series of 24 Patients. *Oral* 2023, *3*, 123–133. https://doi.org/10.3390/oral3010011

Academic Editor: Olga Di Fede

Received: 28 January 2023
Revised: 27 February 2023
Accepted: 10 March 2023
Published: 20 March 2023

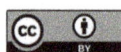

Copyright: © 2023 by the authors. Licensee MDPI, Basel, Switzerland. This article is an open access article distributed under the terms and conditions of the Creative Commons Attribution (CC BY) license (https://creativecommons.org/licenses/by/4.0/).

Abstract: The oral problems of 24 cancer patients on immunotherapy between 2017–2022 and referred by their oncologists, were reported. The age range was 49–80 years, and the median was 64 years. Lung cancer was the most common disease. Three patients a had history of autoimmune disease prior to cancer diagnosis. Patients received immunotherapy for two to 48 months. Prior to immunotherapy, 17 patients received cytotoxic chemotherapy, five angiogenesis inhibitors and one1 radiotherapy to head/neck. During immunotherapy, four patients received chemotherapy, one received bevacizumab, and eight received bone targeting agents, either alone or in combination. Presenting symptoms were oral pain (18 patients, 75%), dental pain (five patients), xerostomia (five patients), burning/itching (seven patients), bleeding (three patients), swelling (three patients), and taste problems (dysgeusia) (three patients). One patient was asymptomatic. Immune-related lesions were observed in 15 patients (62.50%), of which three were exacerbations of prior autoimmune disease. Three patients reported severe deterioration and itching after using a mouthwash. We also observed six (25%) infections (four candidiasis and two herpes simplex), and six (25.00%) cases of medication-related osteonecrosis of the jaw (MRONJ). Five of those MRONJ cases developed among the eight patients with the administration of bone targeting agents and one in a patient with bevacizumab. Two patients presented with more than one lesion. In conclusion, immune-related lesions were most common; oral infections and MRONJ were also observed. Various oral complications might be related to the interplay between immunotherapy and other therapies prior or concurrent to immunotherapy.

Keywords: immunotherapy; cancer; oral toxicities; immune-related oral toxicities; candidiasis; herpes simplex; medication-related osteonecrosis of the jaw

1. Introduction

The use of immune checkpoint inhibitors to treat increasing types of cancers is a revolution in oncology. Immunotherapy blocks the T cell receptor-ligand relationships and restores and activates anti-tumor immunity. It prevents tumors from escaping T cell-mediated killing by inhibiting the biological pathways that would otherwise suppress T cell activation and proliferation [1–5]. This enhanced action against tumor cells may also affect healthy tissues, mounting an immune-related inflammatory reaction with variable clinical presentations. This toxicity in known as immune-related adverse events (irAEs), and differs from standard chemotherapy toxicities due to their immune-related pathogenic mechanism [1–9].

Some patients may already have a history of an autoimmune disease in the mouth or in other body systems. In that case, immunotherapy can exacerbate the prior autoimmune disease of the patient [10–12]. Others on immunotherapy may also receive other antineoplastic medications and may be at risk of complications and toxicities related to those other antineoplastic therapies. The synergistic effects, if any, between immunotherapy and other prior or concurrent anticancer therapies have not been studied. Immunotherapy and irAEs may adversely affect patients' quality of life [13].

Dermatologic and gastrointestinal toxicity, polyarthritis, endocrinopathies, and pneumonitis are the most common irAEs that have been described. [1–9,14–18]. In a recent study which compared durvalumab alone to a combination of Durvalumab, fatigue, diarrhea, hypothyroidism, anemia, and constipation were the most common adverse events. No oral toxicity was reported [19].

The primary treatment strategy for those immune-related toxicities is corticosteroid use, systemic or topical, additional immunosuppression, and treatment interruption or discontinuation [1,10,11,14–18].

Reports on oral toxicities related to immunotherapy are sparse. Some clinical trials and reviews have reported xerostomia as the only oral toxicity in immunotherapy, with an incidence between 3% and 7% [2,6,8,15]. No oral mucosal irAEs have been described in other trials and reviews [1,4,5,7,9].

The oral mucosal irAEs have often been described, in case reports and case series, as "oral lichenoid reactions". The mucous membrane pemphigoid, erythema multiforme, Stevens-Johnson syndrome, and Sjogren syndrome are less commonly reported [15,20–28]. The term "oral mucositis or stomatitis" associated with immunotherapy was used in two case reports and a retrospective study by other medical oncology clinics [29–31]. The term "oral mucosal disorders" was used in an analysis of the oral problems of 317 patients from electronic files [32]. Medication-related osteonecrosis of the jaw (MRONJ) has been recently described, in a few case reports, as an additional toxicity in patients who receive immunotherapies of [33–38].

The different terms which are used to describe oral mucosal immune related toxicity, such as ir-oral lichenoid reactions, or oral mucositis or stomatitis or oral disorders, combined with the lack of reporting of the oral mucosal irAEs in some in clinical trials, point to the difficulties in recognizing and reporting the oral irAEs. At the same time, immunotherapy is increasingly used, combined with other cancer therapies, leading to various other toxicities. The possible synergistic effects on the oral cavity, if any, have not been studied.

The purpose of this manuscript is to report the oral problems/toxicity of 24 cancer patients who received immunotherapy at presentation to the dentist, either as monotherapy or in combination with other cancer therapies.

2. Patients and Methods

Twenty-four cancer patients who received different immunotherapy medications, were referred by their medical oncologists to the private clinic of ONG for oral oncology consultation between the years 2017 and 2022.

Eight patients were referred from public cancer hospitals and 16 were referred from private hospitals. All patients had undergone an oral clinical evaluation by ONG at the private clinic. A smear for Candida species was taken when needed. Panoramic radiographs or Cone Beam Computed Tomography was performed, when needed, by Drs. EG and DG at the private clinic of ONG.

Patients' files were retrospectively assessed, and patients' characteristics and treatments were included in the present series. This assessment was undertaken as a preliminary case series report, within the scope of planning a multicenter research study of oral toxicities of immunotherapy. Oral lesions, treatments, prior and current anticancer therapies, and follow-up information were recorded.

3. Results

There were 19 males and 5 females in the study, with a median age of 64 years. Lung cancer was the most common diagnosis. Eight patients received immunotherapy combined with chemotherapy ($n = 4$), and/or bone targeting agents (BTA, $n = 8$), or an angiogenesis inhibitor (bevacizumab) ($n = 1$). Medications have been described, in detail, in Table 1. Three patients had a history of autoimmune disease prior to cancer diagnosis. One of those cases has been published [28]. Twenty patients had been pretreated with cytotoxic chemotherapy ($n = 17$) and/or angiogenesis inhibitors ($n = 5$), alone or in combination with other therapies.

The reasons for referral included oral pain, dental/mandible pain, burning/itching, bleeding, swelling and taste problems, leading to eating difficulties and dysphagia. One patient, although asymptomatic, was referred by his oncologist after reporting a dental extraction two months prior (Table 2).

Immune-related oral lesions were diagnosed in 15 patients. Twelve were consistent with oral lichenoid reactions (Figure 1), while mucosal bullous formation was clinically consistent with benign mucous membrane pemphigoids in three patients (Figure 2).

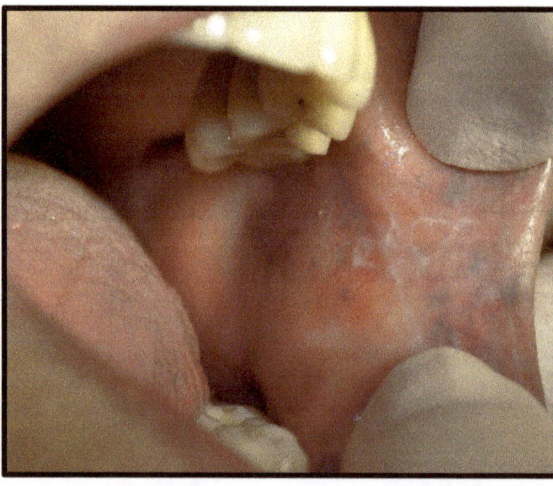

Figure 1. irLichenoid reaction. The patient, on pembrolizumab, presented with oral pain, mild burning/itching, dysphagia, and difficulty in cleaning teeth. White striae are seen on the buccal mucosa.

Table 1. Patients and disease characteristics and medications, $n = 24$.

		n	%
Gender		19/5	79.2/20.8
	M/F		
Age/years			
Range/median	49–80/64		
Mean age/standard deviation	65.88/9.20		
Cancer type			
	Lung ca	15	62.50
	Renal Cell ca	4	16.66
	Melanoma	2	8.33
	Urothelial ca	2	8.33
	Oral ca	1	4.16
Immunotherapy		24	100.00
	Nivolumab	11	
	Pembrolizumab	10	
	Atezolizumab	1	
	Ipilimumab switched to Nivolumab	1	
	Pembrolizumab switched to Ipilimumab	1	
Cancer therapy prior to immunotherapy		20	83.33
	CT alone	14	58.33
	CT+Zoledronic acid	1	4.16
	CT+Bevacizumab	2	8.33
	Angiogenesis inhibitors alone	3	12.50
	Sunitinib, $n = 1$		
	Sunitinib followed by Cabozantinib, $n = 1$		
	Temsirolimus followed by Sunitinib, $n = 1$		
	Radiotherapy to Head/Neck	1	4.16
Therapy concurrent with immunotherapy		9	37.5
	Cytotoxic CT, 1 alone and 3 combined with other drugs	4	16.66
	BTA alone (zol, $n = 2$, Den = 3)	5	20.83
	BTA in combination ($n = 3$), as following	3	12.50
	CT+Bevacizumab+Zoledronic acid	1	
	CT+Zoledronic acid	1	
	CT+Denosumab	1	
Patients with a history of autoimmune disease		3	12.50
	Oral lichen planus & autoimmune biliary cirrhosis	1	
	Dermal lichen planus	1	
	Vitiligo	1	

M = Male, F = Female, CT = Chemotherapy, BTA = Bone Targeting Agent, Zol = zoledronic acid, Den = denosumab.

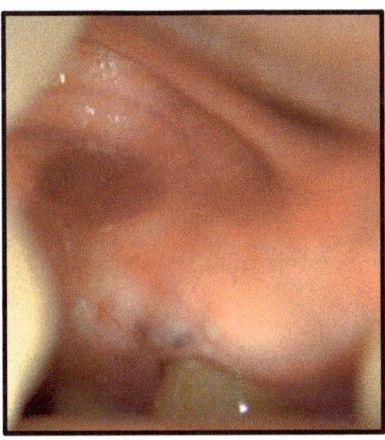

Figure 2. Hemorrhagic blisters, right buccal gingivae, consistent with benign mucous membrane pemphigoid. The patient, on pembrolizumab, presented with pain and dysphagia.

Table 2. Reason for referral, diagnosis of oral lesion and management, $n = 24$.

	n	%
Reason for referral		
Oral pain	18	75.00
Dental/mandible pain	5	20.83
Burning/itching	7	29.16
Xerostomia	5	20.83
Gingival bleeding	3	12.50
Swelling	3	12.50
Taste problems	3	12.50
Dental extraction follow-up	1	4.16
Oral mucosal lesions		
Immune Related	15	62.50
OLP/lichenoid reaction (3 were exacerbations of previous autoimmune disease)	12	50.00
Benign mucous membrane pemphigoid	3	12.50
Management: Costicosteroid mouthwash, with good response		
Infections		
Candidiasis, pseudomembranous (3), & erythematous (1), managed with oral fluconazole	4	16.66
Herpes simplex, lip ulcers, managed with oral acyclovir & topical cream on lip	2	8.33
Osteonecrosis of the mandible, exposed type	6	25.00
Medications with known ONJ risk, prior or concurrent with Immunotherapy		
Prior bevacizumab	1	
Concurrent zoledronic	1	
Prior sunitininb, followed by cabozantinib, concurrent denosumab	1	
Concurrent bevacizumab & zoledronic acid	1	
Prior & concurrent zoledronic acid	1	
Concurrent denosumab	1	
Management: Conservative, antibiotics	6	
Patients with more than one lesion at presentation	2	8.33
Lichenoid reaction+candidiasis+herpes	1	
MRONJ + Candidiasis	1	

OLP = oral lichen planus, ONJ = osteonecrosis of the jaw.

Three patients had lesions which were exacerbations of previous oral and dermal lichen planus, and one had vitiligo. (Figure 3). Three patients presented with painful ulcers following the use of mouthwash (Figure 4). The mouthwash was used to alleviate mild oral mucosal symptoms after the initiation of immunotherapy.

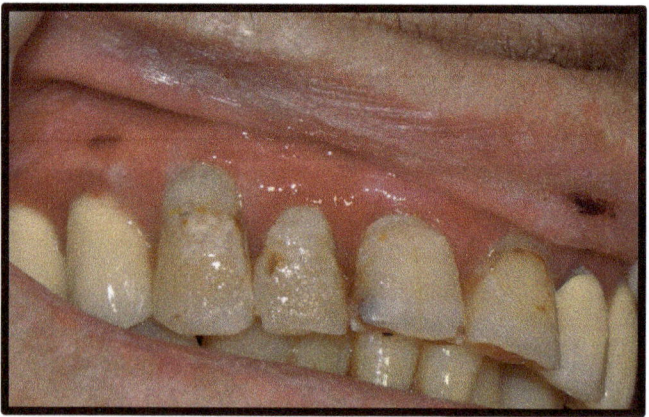

Figure 3. Exacerbation of oral lichen planus; the biopsy was documented years before the cancer diagnosis. The patient, on pembrolizumab and switched to ipilimumab, presented with oral/gingival pain, bleeding, and the inability to perform oral hygiene.

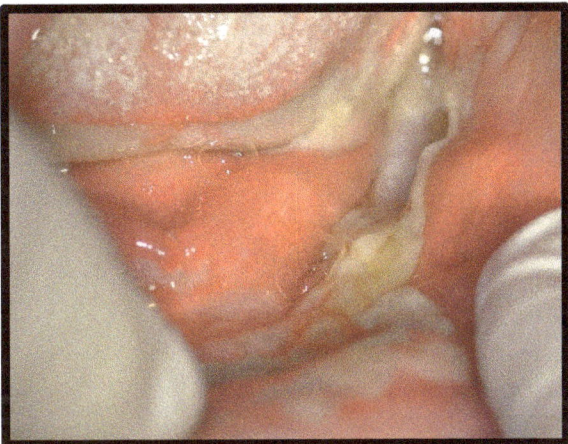

Figure 4. Oral mucosal ulcers on the floor of mouth, the mandible, and the lip mucosa. The patient used itching/burning mouthwash. The patient, on pembrolizumab, presented with severe oral pain.

Six patients had oral infections; four were candidiasis (Figure 5), and two were herpes simplex recurrent infections, presenting as blisters and ulcers, with crusting on the vermillion border and commissures (Figure 6). Five patients reported xerostomia, which was related to oral candidiasis ($n = 3$), an irLichenoid reaction ($n = 1$), and mouthwash use ($n = 1$).

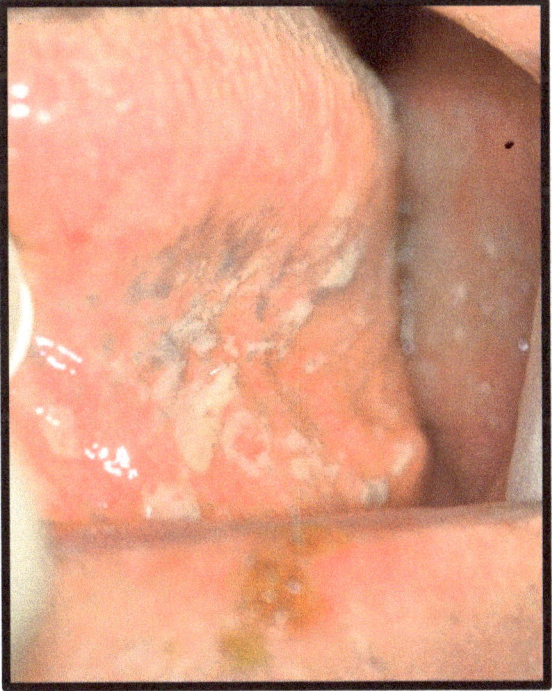

Figure 5. Oral pseudomembranous candidiasis, with positive Candida albicans, on the ventral and lateral tongue. The patient, on pembrolizumab, presented with xerostomia and dysphagia. Herpes labialis was also seen on the lower lip.

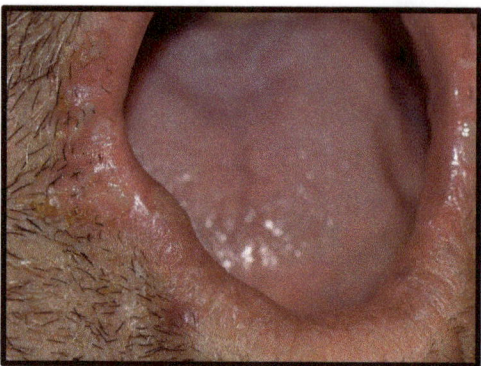

Figure 6. Herpes simplex virus infection on both lip commissures, presenting with blisters and crusting. The patient, on nivolumab, was in pain for more than one month.

MRONJ on the mandible was diagnosed in six patients (Figure 7). Five of those patients had received bone targeting agents during immunotherapy, combined either prior or concurrent with angiogenesis inhibitors, and one had received bevacizumab prior to nivolumab (Table 2). The patient with MRONJ, with prior bevacizumab, was included in our review on MRONJ related to non-antiresorptives [33].

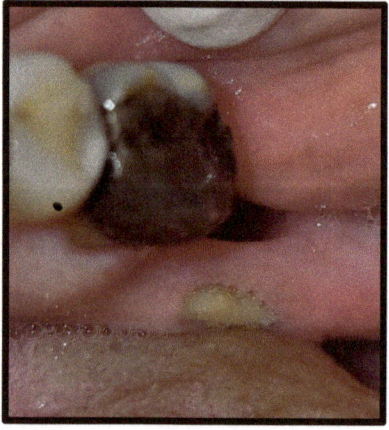

Figure 7. MRONJ, right lingual mandible. The patient, on atezolizumab and zoledronic acid and chemotherapy, presented with pain in the jaw two months after dental extraction due to dental pain.

Two patients presented with more than one oral lesion: one with a lichenoid reaction at first visit and oral candidiasis and herpes labialis at the re-examination one week later, and a second patient presented with MRONJ and oral candidiasis.

The reasons for referral: oral mucosal diseases, MRONJ and medications, are shown in Table 2.

Topical corticosteroids, oral fluconazole, miconazole topical cream and oral and/or topical acyclovir were administered. The patients responded well. Immunotherapy was discontinued in five patients who had irPneumonitis (n = 2), thrombosis (n = 1), irHepatitis (n = 1), and disease progression (n = 1). The BTA was discontinued in all patients, and MRONJ was managed conservatively, since their medical oncologists and the patients themselves did not consent to surgical management.

4. Discussion

Reports on the oral problems in patients who receive immunotherapy are sparse and have been described in patients who have received single agent checkpoint inhibitors [15,22,25,27,32]. However, patients who receive immunotherapy, may have also received other cancer therapies, either prior to or concurrently with immunotherapy.

The oral problems have often been defined as irLichenoid reactions, mucous membrane pemphigoid, and xerostomia. Recently, a few cases of osteonecrosis of the jaw in patients who received immunotherapy either alone or combined with other therapies have been published [33–38]. In the present series, 9 of the 24 patients, while on immunotherapy, received other anticancer or cancer supportive care medications, such as cytotoxic chemotherapy, angiogenesis inhibitors, and/or bone targeting agents. Twenty of our patients were also pretreated with cytotoxic chemotherapy and/or angiogenesis inhibitors or zoledronic acid.

Immune-related lichenoid reactions and mucous membrane pemphigoid were common in our study, and were observed in 15 patients. Most lesions were low-grade and were relieved with topical corticosteroids, as reported by other investigators [21–25,27,28]. Extensive and painful oral ulcerations were attributed to the use of a mouthwash in three patients who reported the worsening of mild oral symptoms following immunotherapy. Mouthwash was introduced following immunotherapy in order to relieve mild oral symptoms.

Oral infections at presentation were diagnosed in six patients. This is the first report of oral infections, as a presenting symptom, in patients who received immunotherapy, although infections are common in the cancer patient setting. Xerostomia, dysgeusia or ageusia and burning were the reasons for referral in patients with oral candidiasis. Oral pain was the presenting symptom in patients with herpes. All six patients responded well to oral and topical antifungal and antiherpetic therapy. Urinary tract infections, pneumonia and sepsis were the most common cause of the discontinuation of immunotherapy in a study of patients who received atezolizumab or pembrolizumab [5]. In another study of 459 dermatology patients with irSkin problems, the authors reported the diagnosis of 24 skin infections [18]. No oral candidiasis or other oral infection or any kind of oral ir problem was observed in any of the above studies [5,18].

Xerostomia was one of the main complaints in five of the patients. It was related with an ir-lichenoid reaction in one patient and with mouthwash use in another patient. Xerostomia was the main complaint in three patients with oral candidiasis. Xerostomia is a risk factor of candidiasis and, on the other hand, xerostomia is one of the first symptoms of oral candidiasis. Michot et al., in their review of immune related adverse events, reported that about 5% of patients who receive an immune checkpoint blockade have symptoms of dry mouth [6]. They recommend, however, that oral candidiasis must be firstly ruled out in this context. Ir-xerostomia has been reported in a small case series and in several clinical trials of immunotherapy, and ranged from 6.0% to 24% [2,6,8,39]. In a review of the electronic medical records of 4683 patients who received immunotherapy, xerostomia was the most common oral disorder (68.5%), followed by oral mucosal disorders (33.4%) and dysgeusia (24.0%) [31]. The authors commented that additional studies are warranted to better characterize oral irAEs and their biologic basis.

Medication related osteonecrosis of the jaw was diagnosed in six patients, all on the mandible and all of the exposed type. Five patients presented with dental pain or pain in the mandible, and one presented with an asymptomatic non-healing post-dental extraction socket. All six patients received medications, with a known risk for MRONJ, such as angiogenesis inhibitors and/or bone targeting agents, either prior to or concurrent with immunotherapy. MRONJ has emerged as another, although rare, oral toxicity in patients on immunotherapy [33–38]. The first report was associated with ipilimumab therapy [33]. Another case was related to nivolumab with the prior administration of bevacizumab, and three more cases of MRONJ were related to pembrolizumab and epacadostat, to nivolumab, and to ipilimumab with the implication of a role for targeted therapy [34–37]. Recently, a case of MRONJ was related to the combined treatment with pembrolizumab and denosumab [38]. The knowledge on the role of immunotherapy in the development of MRONJ, beyond the few case reports, either alone or combined with other medications, with a known risk for osteonecrosis of the jaw, is limited, and it remains to be explored. Xu et al. [32] noted in their study that cytotoxic chemotherapy may exacerbate the risk of oral adverse events. Recently, cytotoxic chemotherapy was found to increase the risk of exacerbations of periodontitis [40], while dental/periodontal infection is the most important local risk factor for MRONJ [41]. Furthermore, the dental/periodontal infection, when associated with histologically necrotic periodontal bone, may be an early stage of MRONJ [42–44].

Twenty of the 24 patients in the present study, had been pretreated with cytotoxic chemotherapy and/or angiogenesis inhibitors or a BTA prior to immunotherapy. Four patients were receiving chemotherapy at presentation, concurrently with immunotherapy, while eight were receiving bone targeting agents; four patients were receiving zoledronic acid and four were receiving denosumab.

In conclusion, oral mucosal irAEs were observed in 15 of a series of 24 patients on immunotherapy, who were referred by their oncologists for different oral symptoms. Furthermore, six oral mucosal infections and six MRONJ cases were observed.

The rapidly increasing use of immunotherapy, the increasing types of cancers treated with immunotherapy, and the need for therapy combinations, in the real world, highlight the necessity for physician awareness of the potential for oral irAEs. Prospective studies should examine the possible synergistic effects of therapy combinations on the oral mucosa. Educational programs may help raise awareness and improve the communication between the members of the multidisciplinary team, resulting in the timely and successful management of the patient.

Author Contributions: O.N.-G., E.G. and D.G. examined the patients, diagnosed the oral problems, and wrote the manuscript. A.P., N.T., H.L., I.A., D.K., E.R., N.K. (Nikolaos Katirtzoglou), N.K. (Nikolaos Kentepozidis), P.K., F.S., E.K., D.D., G.T., G.M., S.K., P.G. and K.S. referred the patients and read, edited, and approved the manuscript. All authors have read and agreed to the published version of the manuscript.

Funding: This research received no external funding.

Institutional Review Board Statement: Not applicable.

Informed Consent Statement: Written informed consent form was obtained by all patients whose clinical photos are included in the manuscript.

Data Availability Statement: Not applicable.

Conflicts of Interest: The authors declare that they have no conflict of interest.

References

1. Fecher, L.A.; Agarwala, S.S.; Hodi, F.S.; Weber, J.S. Ipilimumab and its toxicities: A multidisciplinary approach. *Oncologist* **2013**, *18*, 733–743. [CrossRef] [PubMed]
2. Topalian, S.L.; Sznol, M.; McDermott, D.F.; Kluger, H.M.; Carvajal, R.D.; Sharfman, W.H.; Brahmer, J.R.; Lawrence, D.P.; Atkins, M.B.; Powderly, J.D.; et al. Survival, durable tumor response, and long-term safety in patients with advanced melanoma receiving nivolumab. *J. Clin. Oncol.* **2014**, *32*, 1020–1031. [CrossRef] [PubMed]
3. Ling, D.C.; Bakkenist, C.J.; Ferris, R.L.; Clump, D.C. Role of immunotherapy in head and neck cancer. *Sem. Radiat. Oncol.* **2017**, *28*, 12–16. [CrossRef]
4. Larkins, E.; Blumenthal, G.M.; Yuan, W.; He, K.; Sridhara, R.; Subramanian, S.; Zhao, H.; Liu, C.; Yu, J.; Goldberg, K.B.; et al. FDA approval summary: Pembrolizumab for the treatment of recurrent or metastatic head and neck squamous cell carcinoma with disease progression on or after platinum-containing chemotherapy. *Oncologist* **2017**, *22*, 873–878. [CrossRef] [PubMed]
5. Suzman, D.L.; Agrawal, S.; Ning, Y.-M.; Maher, E.; Fernandes, L.L.; Karuri, S.; Tang, S.; Sridhara, R.; Schroeder, J.; Goldberg, K.B.; et al. FDA approval summary: Atezolizumab or pembrolizumab for the treatment of patients with advanced urothelial carcinoma ineligible for cisplatin-containing chemotherapy. *Oncologist* **2019**, *24*, 563–569. [CrossRef] [PubMed]
6. Michot, J.M.; Bigenwald, C.; Champiat, S.; Collins, M.; Carbonnel, F.; Postel-Vinay, S.; Beldelou, A.; Varga, A.; Bahleda, R.; Hollebecque, A.; et al. Immune related adverse events with immune checkpoint blockade: A comprehensive review. *Eur. J. Cancer* **2016**, *54*, 139–148. [CrossRef] [PubMed]

7. Wang, P.F.; Chen, Y.; Song, S.Y.; Wang, T.J.; Ji, W.J.; Li, S.W.; Liu, N.; Yan, C.-X. Immune-related adverse events associated with anti-PD-1/PD-L1 treatment for malignancies: A meta-analysis. *Front. Oncol.* **2017**, *8*, 730. [CrossRef]
8. Kennedy, L.B.; Salama, A.H.K.S. A review of cancer immunotherapy toxicity. *CA Cancer J. Clin.* **2020**, *70*, 86–104. [CrossRef]
9. Gumusay, O.; Callan, J.; Rugo, H.S. Immunotherapy toxicity: Identification and management. *Breast Cancer Res. Treat.* **2022**, *192*, 1–17. [CrossRef]
10. Johnson, D.B.; Sullivan, R.J.; Ott, P.A.; Carlino, M.S.; Khushalani, N.I.; Ye, F.; Guminski, A.; Puzanov, I.; Lawrence, D.P.; Buchbinder, E.I.; et al. Ipilimumab therapy in patients with advanced melanoma and preexisting autoimmune disorders. *JAMA Oncol.* **2016**, *2*, 234–240. [CrossRef]
11. Danlos, F.-X.; Voisin, A.-L.; Dyevre, V.; Michot, J.-M.; Routier, E.; Taillade, L.; Champiat, S.; Aspeslagh, S.; Haroche, J.; Albiges, L.; et al. Safety and efficacy of anti-programmed death 1 antibodies in patients with cancer and pre-existing autoimmune or inflammatory disease. *Eur. J. Cancer* **2018**, *91*, 21–29. [CrossRef] [PubMed]
12. Ijaz, A.; Khan, A.Y.; Malik, S.U.; Faridi, W.; Fraz, M.A.; Usman, M.; Tariq, M.J.; Durer, S.; Durer, C.; Russ, A.; et al. Significant risk of graft-versus-host disease with exposure to checkpoint inhibitors before and after allogeneic transplantation. *Biol. Blood Marrow Transpl.* **2018**, *25*, 94–99. [CrossRef] [PubMed]
13. O'Reilly, A.; Hughes, P.; Mann, J.; Zhuangming, L.; Teh, J.J.; Mclean, E.; Edmonds, K.; Lingard, K.; Chauhan, D.; Lynch, J.; et al. An immunotherapy survivor population: Health-related quality of life and toxicity in patients with metastatic melanoma treated with immune checkpoint inhibitors. *Support. Care Cancer* **2020**, *28*, 561–570. [CrossRef]
14. Sundaresan, S.B.A.; Nguyen, K.T.; Nelson, K.C.; Ivan, D.; Patel, A.B. Erythema multiforme major in a patient with metastatic melanoma treated with nivolumab. *Dermatol. Online J.* **2017**, *23*, 1–3. [CrossRef]
15. Rapoport, B.L.; van Eeden, R.; Sibaud, V.; Epstein, J.B.; Klastersky, J.; Aapro, M.; Moodley, D. Supportive care for patients undergoing immunotherapy. *Support. Care Cancer* **2017**, *25*, 3017–3030. [CrossRef] [PubMed]
16. Saw, S.; Yueh, H.; Ng, Q.S. Pembrolizumab-induced Stevens-Johnson syndrome in non-melanoma patients. *Eur. J. Cancer* **2017**, *81*, 237–239. [CrossRef]
17. Salati, M.; Pifferi, M.; Baldessari, C.; Bertolini, F.; Tomasello, C.; Cascinu, S.; Barbieri, F. Stevens-Johnson syndrome during nivolumab treatment of NSCLC. *Ann. Oncol.* **2018**, *29*, 283–284. [CrossRef]
18. Nikolaou, V.; Voudouri, D.; Tsironis, G.; Charpidou, A.; Stamoulis, G.; Triantafyllopoulou, I.; Panoutsopoulou, I.; Xidakis, E.; Bamias, A.; Samantas, E. Cutaneous toxicities of antineoplastic agents: Data from a large cohort of Greek patients. *Support. Care Cancer* **2019**, *27*, 4535–4542. [CrossRef]
19. Psyrri, A.; Harrington, K.; Gillison, M.; Ahn, M.J.; Takahashi, S.; Weiss, J.; Machiels, J.P.; Vasilyev, H.; Karpenko, A. Durvalumab with or without tremelimumab versus the EXTREME regimen, as first-line treatment for recurrent or metastatic squamous cell carcinoma of the head and neck: KESTREL, a randomized, open-label, phase III study. *Ann. Oncol.* **2023**, *34*, 263–274. [CrossRef]
20. Jackson, L.K.; Johnson, D.B.; Sosman, J.A.; Murphy, B.A.; Epstein, J.B. Oral health in oncology: Impact of immunotherapy. *Support. Care Cancer* **2015**, *23*, 1–3. [CrossRef]
21. Lacouture, M.; Sibeaud, V. Toxic side effects of targeted therapies and immunotherapies affecting the skin, oral mucosa, hair, and nails. *Am. J. Dermatol.* **2018**, *19*, S31–S39. [CrossRef] [PubMed]
22. Sibaud, V.; Eid, C.; Belum, V.R.; Combemale, P.; Barres, B.; Lamant, L.; Mourey, L.; Gomez-Roca, C.; Estilo, C.L.; Motzer, R.; et al. Oral lichenoid reactions associated with anti-PD-1/PD-L1 therapies: Clinicopathological findings. *J. Eur. Acad. Dermatol. Venerol.* **2017**, *31*, e464–e469. [CrossRef] [PubMed]
23. Klein, B.A.; Shazib, M.A.; Villa, A.; Alves, F.d.A.; Vacharotayangul, P.; Sonis, S.; Fedele, S.; Treister, N.S. Immune checkpoint inhibitors in cancer therapy: Review of orofacial adverse events and role of the oral healthcare provider. *Front. Oral Health* **2022**, *3*, 83. [CrossRef]
24. Klein, B.A.; Alves, F.A.; Velho, J.D.S.R.; Vachrotayangul, P.; Hanna, G.J.; LeBoeuf, N.R.; Shazib, M.A.; Villa, A.; Woo, S.B.; Sroussi, H.; et al. Oral manifestations of immune-related adverse events in cancer patients treated with immune checkpoint inhibitors. *Oral Dis.* **2021**, *28*, 9–22. [CrossRef] [PubMed]
25. Obara, K.; Masuzawa, M.; Amoh, Y. Oral lichenoid reaction showing multiple ulcers associated with anti-programmed death cell receptor-1 treatment: A report of two cases and published work review. *J. Dermatol.* **2018**, *45*, 587–591. [CrossRef] [PubMed]
26. Bhattacharyya, I.; Chehal, H.; Migliorati, C. Severe oral erosive lichenoid reaction to pembrolizumab therapy. *Oral Surg. Oral Med. Oral Pathol.* **2020**, *130*, e301–e307. [CrossRef]
27. Shazib, M.A.; Woo, S.B.; Sroussi, H.; Carvo, I.; Treister, N.; Farag, A.; Schoenfeld, J.; Haddad, R.; LeBoeuf, N.; Villa, A. Oral immune-related adverse events associated with PD-1 inhibitor therapy: A case series. *Oral Dis.* **2020**, *26*, 325–333. [CrossRef]
28. Economopoulou, P.; Nicolatou-Galitis, O.; Kotsantis, I.; Psyrri, A. Nivolumab-related lichen planus of the lip in a patient with head and neck cancer. *Oral Oncol.* **2020**, *104*, 104623. [CrossRef]
29. Yoon, S.Y.; Han, J.J.; Baek, S.K.; Kim, H.J.; Maeng, C.H. Pembrolizumab-induced severe oral mucositis in a patient with squamous cell carcinoma of the lung: A case study. *Lung Cancer* **2020**, *147*, 21–25. [CrossRef]
30. Sheth, H.; Pragya, R.; Kovale, S.; Deshpande, M.; Mistry, R.; Shreenivas, A.; Limaye, S. Oral mucositis-case series of a rare adverse effect associated with immunotherapy. *Support. Care Cancer* **2021**, *29*, 4705–4709. [CrossRef]
31. Jacob, J.S.; Dutra, B.E.; Garcia-Rodriguez, V.; Panneerselvan, K.; Abraham, A.; Zou, F.; Ma, W.; Grivas, P.; Thompson, J.A.; Altan, M.; et al. Clinical characteristics and outcomes of oral mucositis associated with immune checkpoint inhibitors in patients with cancer. *J. Natl. Compr. Cancer Netw.* **2021**, *12*, 1415–1424. [CrossRef] [PubMed]

32. Xu, Y.; Wen, N.; Sonis, S.T.; Villa, A. Oral side effects of immune checkpoint inhibitor therapy (ICIT): An analysis of 4683 patients receiving ICIT for malignancies at Massachusetts General Hospital, Brigham & Women's Hospital, and the Dana-Farber Cancer Institute, 2011 to 2019. *Cancer* **2021**, *127*, 1796–1804. [CrossRef] [PubMed]
33. Owosho, A.A.; Scordo, M.; Yom, S.K.; Randazzo, J.; Chapman, P.B.; Huryn, J.M.; Estilo, C.L. Osteonecrosis of the jaw a new complication related to ipilimumab. *Oral Oncol.* **2015**, *51*, e100–e101. [CrossRef] [PubMed]
34. Nicolatou-Galitis, O.; Kouri, M.; Papadopoulou, E.; Vardas, E.; Galiti, D.; Epstein, J.B.; Elad, S.; Campisi, G.; Tsoukalas, N.; Bektas-Kayhan, K.; et al. Osteonecrosis of the jaw related to non-antiresorptive medications: A systematic review. *Support. Care Cancer* **2019**, *27*, 383–394. [CrossRef]
35. Decaux, J.; Magremanne, M. Medication-related osteonecrosis of the jaw related to epacadostat and pembrolizumab. *J. Stomatol. Oral Maxillofac Surg.* **2020**, *121*, 740–742. [CrossRef] [PubMed]
36. Pundole, X.; Jones, A.L.; Tetzlaff, M.T.; Williams, M.D.; Murphy, W.A., Jr.; Otun, A.; Goepfert, R.P.; Davies, M.A. Osteonecrosis of the jaw induced by treatment with anti-PD-1 immunotherapy: A case report. *Immunotherapy* **2020**, *12*, 1213–1219. [CrossRef] [PubMed]
37. Guida, A.; Perri, F.; Ionna, F.; Ascierto, P.A.; Grimaldi, A.M. New-generation anticancer drugs and medication-related osteonecrosis of the jaw (MRONJ): Late onset 3 years after ipilimumab endovenous administration with a possible role of target therapy. *Clin. Case Rep.* **2021**, *9*, 61–66. [CrossRef]
38. Myoken, Y.; Fujita, Y.; Kawamoto, K.; Toratani, S. Osteonecrosis of the jaw in a metastatic lung cancer patient with bone metastases undergoing pembrolizumab + denosumab combination therapy: Case report and literature review. *Oral Oncol.* **2020**, *111*, 104874. [CrossRef]
39. Bustillos, H.; Indorf, A.; Alwan, L.; Thompson, J.; Jung, L. Xerostomia: An immunotherapy-related adverse effect in cancer patients. *Support. Care Cancer* **2022**, *30*, 1681–1687. [CrossRef]
40. Villafluerte, K.R.V.; Taba, M., Jr.; Messora, M.; Dos Reis, F.J.C.; Carrara, H.A.; Martinez, C.d.J.H.; Palioto, D.B. Effects of non-surgical periodontal therapy on the cytokine profile in gingival crevicular fluid of breast cancer patients with periodontitis undergoing chemotherapy. *Support. Care Cancer* **2021**, *29*, 7505–7513. [CrossRef]
41. Schiodt, M.; Otto, S.; Fedele, S.; Bedogni, A.; Nicolatou-Galitis, O.; Guggenberger, R.; Brokstad Herlofson, B.; Ristow, O.; Kofod, T. Workshop of European Task force on medication-related osteonecrosis of the jaw-Current challenges. *Oral Dis.* **2019**, *25*, 1815–1821. [CrossRef] [PubMed]
42. Nicolatou-Galitis, O.; Papadopoulou, L.E.; Vardas, E.; Kouri, M.; Galiti, D.; Galitis, E.; Alexiou, K.E.; Tsiklakis, K.; Ardavanis, A.; Razis, E.; et al. Alveolar bone histological nexcrosis observed prior to extractions in patients, who receive bone-targeting agents. *Oral Dis.* **2020**, *26*, 955–966. [CrossRef] [PubMed]
43. Ristow, O.; Rückschloß, T.; Moratin, J.; Müller, M.; Kühle, R.; Dominik, H.; Pliz, M.; Shavlokhova, V.; Otto, S.; Hoffman, J.; et al. Wound closure and alveoloplasty after preventive tooth extractions in patients with antiresorptive intake-A randomized pilot study. *Oral Dis.* **2021**, *27*, 532–546. [CrossRef] [PubMed]
44. Otto, S.; Aljohani, S.; Fleifel, R.; Ecke, S.; Ristow, O.; Burian, E.; Troeltzsch, M.; Pauke, C.; Ehrenfeld, M. Infection as an important factor in Medication-Related Osteonecrosis of the Jaw (MRONJ). *Medicina* **2021**, *57*, 463. [CrossRef]

Disclaimer/Publisher's Note: The statements, opinions and data contained in all publications are solely those of the individual author(s) and contributor(s) and not of MDPI and/or the editor(s). MDPI and/or the editor(s) disclaim responsibility for any injury to people or property resulting from any ideas, methods, instructions or products referred to in the content.

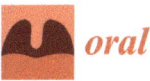 *oral*

Review

Protection of Patient Data in Digital Oral and General Health Care: A Scoping Review with Respect to the Current Regulations

Olga Di Fede [1,†], Gaetano La Mantia [1,2,3,*,†], Mario G. C. A. Cimino [4] and Giuseppina Campisi [1,2]

1 Department Di.Chir.On.S., University of Palermo, 90127 Palermo, Italy
2 Unit of Oral Medicine and Dentistry for Fragile Patients, Department of Rehabilitation, Fragility, and Continuity of Care, University Hospital Palermo, 90127 Palermo, Italy
3 Department of Biomedical and Dental Sciences and Morphofunctional Imaging, University of Messina, 98147 Messina, Italy
4 Department of Information Engineering, University of Pisa, 56122 Pisa, Italy
* Correspondence: gaetano.lamantia@community.unipa.it
† These authors contributed equally to this work.

Abstract: The use of digital health technologies, including telemedicine and teledentistry, has become a necessity in healthcare due to the SARS-CoV-19 pandemic. These technologies allow for the reduction of the workload of healthcare providers and the improvement of patient outcomes in cases of remote monitoring, diagnosis, and communication. While there are no doubtful benefits, there are some counterparts, such as concerns about clinical risks, data security, and privacy protection. This paper aims to review the regulations regarding the use of digital health apps and software in healthcare. This scoping review followed the PRISMA-ScR guidelines and the five-step framework of Arksey and O'Malley. Study selection was based on eligibility criteria that were defined using the population-exposure framework. The review of the articles selected (*n* = 24) found that the majority focused on data security policies in the healthcare industry, highlighting the need for comprehensive regulations and app control systems to protect patient data. The articles also emphasized the requirement for more appropriate research and policy initiatives to improve data security practices and better address privacy and safety challenges related to health-related apps. The review recognized that papers did not report consistent standards in professional obligation and informed consent in online medical consultations, with potential risks for data privacy, medical liabilities, and ethical issues. Digital health has already revolutionized medical service delivery through technology but faces some challenges, including the lack of standardized protocols for handling sensitive patient data and the absence of common legislative provisions, raising concerns about confidentiality and security. To address these issues and deficiencies, regulatory compliance is crucial to clarify and harmonize regulations and provide guidelines for doctors and the health system. In conclusion, regulating patient data, clarifying provisions, and addressing informed patients are critical and urgent steps in maximizing usage and successful implementation of telemedicine.

Keywords: social app; WhatsApp; GDPR; HIPAA; sensitive data; mobile health; secure messaging app; COVID; dentistry

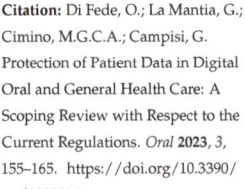

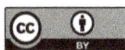

1. Introduction

A rapid transition to digital health technologies is becoming effective in all medical fields [1], and e-health is considered a solution to safely provide care to patients and ensure continuous health care even at a distance [2]. The SARS-CoV-19 pandemic of recent years has accelerated all aspects of health care, including oral health care [3]. In particular, conventional dentistry was reduced and, in some cases, interrupted to minimize the risk of exposure to the SARS-CoV-19 virus for both practitioners and patients by avoiding in-person visits. Health and dental care organizations had to propose and plan alternative protocols [1,4–6].

Telemedicine and teledentistry are used to support clinicians and patients by providing remote monitoring services, remote diagnosis, counseling, home care, and education with self-care management [7–9]; at the same time, they are useful in reducing the workload of health care providers, simplifying interprofessional communication, providing an easy way to share patient information, and giving remote instructions [10–12].

Telemedicine has revolutionized healthcare by providing patients with convenient and accessible medical services. With the help of wireless patient monitoring devices, smartphones, personal digital assistants, and tablets, patients can now connect with specialists in real-time [13]. This eliminates the need for physical visits to the hospital, reducing lost time and allowing for quicker diagnoses. The feedback system in telemedicine also allows for continuous monitoring of the patient's health status, enabling healthcare providers to track any changes and respond promptly. This proactive approach to health management aims to improve outcomes and reduce health risks.

Moreover, telemedicine promotes informed decision-making by giving patients access to their health data and enabling them to actively participate in their own care. This can result in increased patient engagement and improved health outcomes as patients are empowered to make informed choices about their health and take action to maintain good health [9,14,15].

Social media platforms, including WhatsApp, have become an integral part of modern life, with almost half of the world's population using them [16]. As a result, healthcare professionals have adopted these platforms in their daily work to communicate and share information with their peers and patients [17–22]. While there is some evidence to suggest that using social media in healthcare can have many benefits, such as improved communication and data transfer, there are also concerns about the risks associated with its use [21,23–25].

One of the main risks is the potential for breaches of patient privacy and confidentiality. Social media platforms are public forums, and patient information shared on these platforms can be easily accessed by individuals who are not authorized to view it. In addition, patients may inadvertently disclose sensitive health information on social media, compromising their privacy and putting them at risk for discrimination or other negative consequences [26].

There is a lack of consensus in the scientific literature regarding the use of social media in healthcare, with some studies highlighting its positive aspects while others focus on the negative consequences, including clinical risks to patients, data security, and privacy protection. In addition, the use of generic apps and software to exchange health data indiscriminately is not allowed, as it poses a threat to patient safety and data security [27–32]. Given these conflicting views, this paper aims to perform a scoping review of the existing literature on regulations and guidelines for telemedicine apps and software and their use among patients and specialists [33,34]. The goal of this review is to analyze all papers on the current regulatory state and issues of telemedicine and identify crucial points to be solved by further research and development.

2. Materials and Methods

A review of the recent literature (years 2020–2022) was conducted, focusing on telemedicine apps and software for health care and the current regulations of digital health data. This initial search revealed 190 publications from January 2020 to December 2022. This scoping review followed Preferred Reporting Items for Systematic Reviews and Meta-Analysis-Scoping Review (PRISMA-ScR) guidelines and Arksey and O'Malley's five-stage framework to identify available evidence [33]. Five iterative stages were involved in the review: (i) Identifying the research question, (ii) identifying relevant studies, (iii) selecting relevant studies, (iv) charting the data, and (v) summarizing results.

2.1. Eligibility Criteria

We included studies that took place between January 2020 and December 2022 and were solely focused on the use of mobile applications and software in healthcare. The review included all aspects of healthcare, including dental, nursing, and rehabilitation.

2.2. Study Selection

Studies were identified by electronic searches of scientific articles from different biomedical databases (i.e., Scopus, PubMed, and Medline). To minimize biases, publications were examined individually by two reviewers (GLM and ODF).

2.3. Search Strategy

The following search terms were used separately and in combination: social app, teledentistry, telehealth, telemedicine, privacy, policy, legacy issues, liability issues, using medical subject headings, and free text. The full-text screening was performed only by the first author, as is common when scoping reviews are conducted [34]. Our screening procedure was guided by defined inclusion and exclusion criteria developed using the population-exposure framework (PEO) (Table 1). Any disagreements were handled by a mutual conversation among authors. Duplicate papers were deleted, after which there was further scrutiny in order to assess their eligibility.

Table 1. Population-Exposure Framework (PEO).

	Inclusion	Exclusion
Population	- Mobile apps and software used in healthcare for telemedicine services - All medical fields	- Mobile apps and software used in health care for research and evaluation and the continuing education of health care providers
Exposure	- Studies focusing on the regulations, privacy policy, data security, and legacy issues of telemedicine services	- Studies not concerned with regulations, privacy policies, data security, or legacy issues of telemedicine services
Outcome	- Studies reporting on the use of social apps and software for telemedicine and related regulation	
Time	- Published from January 2020 to December 2022.	
Study type	- Primary, peer-reviewed research - Full text available	
Language	- English	- Languages other than English

3. Results

The review was conducted in accordance with the Preferred Reporting Items for Systematic Reviews and the Meta-Analysis-Scoping Review (PRISMA-ScR) guidelines to ensure a transparent and comprehensive evaluation of the available literature (Figure 1).

The results of this analysis suggest that a total of 290 records were identified in the databases (Table 2). No duplicate records were removed prior to screening, indicating that the database search was thorough. However, 45 records were flagged as ineligible by the automation tools, indicating that some records did not meet the initial inclusion criteria. After screening, the number of records was reduced to 245. This reduction was likely due to the application of additional inclusion and exclusion criteria that were more specific than the original criteria. In addition, 55 records were excluded, indicating that some records did not meet the additional inclusion and exclusion criteria. Of the 190 records that were screened for eligibility, some reports were excluded for reasons such as the unavailability of full text or being written in a non-English language. These exclusion criteria have been established to ensure that the studies are easily accessible and can be effectively reviewed by the research team. After conducting a systematic search of multiple databases, we included 24 articles out of 290 for analysis.

Table 2. Summary of 24 studies, from 2020 to 2022, regarding the protection of patient data in Digital Health.

Author (Year)	Country	Design of Study	Issues
Agarwal et al., 2020 [35]	India	Research article	Data security policies Privacy policies
Benjumea et al., 2020 [36]	Spain	Review article	Data security policies Privacy policies
Caetano et al., 2020 [37]	Brasil	Research article	Data security policies Privacy policies
Ghosh et al., 2020 [38]	India	Research article	Data security policies Privacy policies Legacy liabilities
Kaplan 2020b [39]	USA	Review article	Data security policies
Mahtta et al., 2021 [40]	USA	Research article	Data security policies
Kichloo et al., 2020 [41]	USA	Review article	Data security policies
Moura et al., 2020 [42]	Portugal	Research article	Data security policies
Gowda et al., 2021 [43]	USA	Research article	Data security policies
Hoaglin et al., 2021 [44]	USA	Research article	Data security policies Legacy liabilities
Pool et al., 2021 [45]	Australia	Review article	Data security policies Privacy policies Legacy liabilities
Tangari et al., 2021 [46]	Australia	Research article	Data security policies Privacy policies
Alfawzan et al., 2022 [47]	Zurich	Review article	Data security policies Privacy policies
Essén et al., 2022 [48]	Sweden	Research article	Data security policies Privacy policies Legacy liabilities
Grundy 2022 [49]	Canada	Review article	Data security policies Privacy policies Legacy liabilities
Maaß et al., 2022 [15]	Germany	Overview article	Data security policies Privacy policies Legacy liabilities
Mazzuca et al., 2022 [50]	Italy	Review article	Data security policies Privacy policies Legacy liabilities
Sujarwoto et al., 2022 [51]	Indonesia	Overview article	Data security policies Privacy policies
Venkatesh et al., 2022 [52]	India	Research article	Data security policies Privacy policies
Eisenstein et al., 2020 [53]	Brasil	Review article	Privacy policies
Perez-Noboa et al., 2021 [54]	Ecuador	Research article	Privacy policies
Wang et al., 2020 [55]	USA	Research article	Legacy liabilities
Lee et al., 2021 [56]	China	Research article	Legacy liabilities
Ferorelli et al., 2022 [57]	Italia	Review article	Legacy liabilities

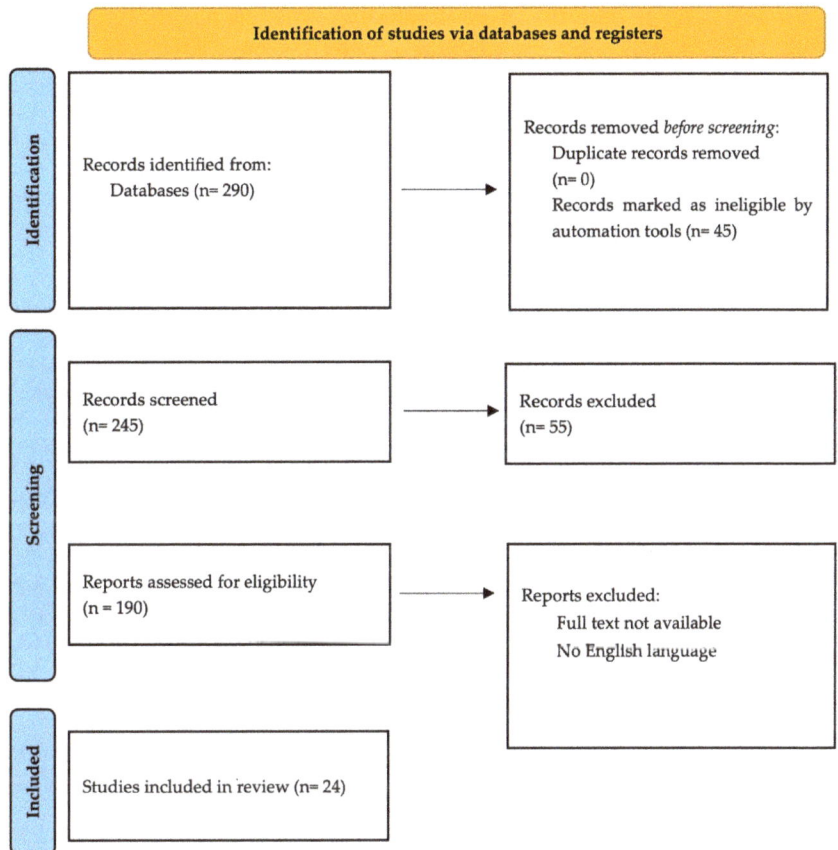

Figure 1. PRISMA flow diagram for systematic reviews.

Through the analysis of these 24 articles, three key themes emerged as crucial components of health app regulations: privacy policies, data security policies, and legacy liabilities. Privacy policies focus on the protection of personal information and sensitive data collected and stored by health apps, while data security policies address the measures in place to secure this information from unauthorized accesses and breaches. Legacy liabilities pertain to the legal responsibilities and obligations of health apps, particularly regarding medical information and advice provided to users. These findings highlight the importance of considering privacy, data security, and legacy liabilities in the regulation of digital health, which is rapidly becoming a popular tool for managing health and wellness.

3.1. Data Security Policies

Data security is a critical issue in the healthcare industry. The need for comprehensive policies and regulations is well documented in the literature. A review of 24 articles revealed that 19 [15,35–45,47–52,58] of them focused on the topic of data security policies, with a specific emphasis on the challenges faced in protecting patient data. The articles pointed out that the lack of comprehensive regulation was a major concern and that the need for an app control system was crucial in preventing the sharing of patient data with unauthorized third parties.

The majority of the articles also emphasized the need for more research in this area, particularly to address the growing concerns around data privacy and security. They suggested that awareness and initiatives by healthcare professionals, healthcare users, and decision-makers were essential in promoting better data security practices. This is especially true in European and American nations that follow GDPR and HIPAA regulations, respectively.

Overall, the findings of these articles highlight the importance of ensuring that patient data is protected and that appropriate policies and regulations are in place to prevent unauthorized access to and sharing of sensitive information. The need for further research, awareness, and initiatives by various stakeholders in the healthcare industry cannot be overemphasized, as data security is critical to protecting the privacy and well-being of patients.

3.2. Privacy Policies

Health-related app policies have been widely discussed in the academic literature, with 15 [15,35–38,45–54] out of 24 articles specifically covering this topic. The studies analyzed the policies in several countries, such as India, Spain, Australia, Zurich, Canada, Brazil, Sweden, Germany, and Italy, and identified challenges related to safety and privacy. These challenges highlight the need for more robust regulations in the areas of operationalization, implementation, and international transferability of approvals.

The lack of proper regulations has been identified as a significant barrier to the widespread adoption and safe utilization of telemedicine platforms, despite their potential benefits, such as improving access to health services and reducing healthcare costs.

The studies suggest that more work is needed in the area of health-related app policies to ensure that telemedicine platforms can be effectively and safely used by people around the world. The regulation of telemedicine is a complex issue that requires cross-national collaboration and commitment to ensuring that these technologies are used to improve health outcomes.

3.3. Professional Legacy Liabilities

The study of 24 articles on online medical consultations revealed that 10 articles [15,38,44,45,48–50,55–57] addressed the issue of liability and legacy concerns. These articles highlighted the risks associated with informed consent, data privacy, medical negligence, and ethical issues in the context of virtual consultations.

The articles discussed the potential risks and challenges associated with providing medical services through online consultations. One of the major issues identified was the need for clear and consistent standards regarding professional liability for medical practitioners who offer online consultations. This is important as the liability issues that arise from online consultations may be different from those associated with traditional face-to-face consultations.

Informed consent was also a weakness in online consultations, as patients may not fully understand the risks and limitations of online medical services. The security of health data was also a concern, as the transmission of sensitive information over the internet could result in data breaches or unauthorized accesses. Medical negligence was another issue raised in the articles selected. The risk of medical malpractice in online consultations is significant, as medical practitioners may not be able to accurately diagnose or treat patients without physically examining them. There is also a potential for ethical issues to arise in online consultations, such as the confidentiality of medical information and the autonomy of patients. Therefore, the articles emphasized the importance of harmonizing the different laws and regulations across different jurisdictions in order to establish a uniform standard for professional liability in online consultations. This will ensure that medical practitioners are held accountable for their actions and that patients are protected from potential harm.

4. Discussion

The review of current regulations on patient data protection in digital oral and general health found several outcomes in privacy policies, data security, and legacy liabilities, in particular, the lack of comprehensive regulations in Europe and America. To improve digital health, there is a need to build secure and adaptable access control models. Awareness should be raised among users, clinicians, developers, and policy makers to carefully consider the benefits and security issues of digital health. Updating guidelines for the ethical use of telemedicine is also necessary to optimize its use and ensure evidence-based practices.

Digital health reduces health disparities and improves access to care through remote screening, treatment, and monitoring. Advanced countries that are investing in digital health include the US, UK, Singapore, South Korea, Sweden, Japan, Australia, Canada, and Germany. To maximize impact, security concerns must be addressed through robust access control models that are widely used in technology. All stakeholders, including users, healthcare providers, tech developers, and policymakers, must consider the security and benefits of mHealth apps.

To enhance its impact, it could be decisive to develop flexible, robust, and risk-conscious access control models for widely used technologies. All stakeholders, including app users, healthcare providers, technology developers, and policymakers, should acknowledge and address security concerns while considering the benefits of mobile health (mHealth) apps [39,44,48,50,51,54].

The review highlights the need for enhancing healthcare providers' care services and raising public awareness on digital health to optimize its benefits. Additionally, updated guidelines for the ethical use of telemedicine and telehealth are required for physicians and organizations [41,52].

Protecting patient data in digital health care is a crucial challenge, since sensitive personal information must remain confidential and secure at all times. Regulations such as the Health Insurance Portability and Accountability Act (HIPAA) in the US and the General Data Protection Regulation (GDPR) in the EU define standards for collecting, storing, and utilizing patient data in digital healthcare [45,59].

Health care providers and organizations must implement appropriate technical and organizational measures, such as encryption and secure backups, and undergo regular security audits to secure patient data from unauthorized access, disclosure, alteration, and destruction as mandated by these regulations [60]. Telemedicine providers must also obtain patient consent for the collection and use of their data and inform patients of their rights under the GDPR and HIPAA. Additionally, patients have the right to access, correct, and delete their personal data and also have to provide their consent for their data to be used for specific purposes. Compliance with these regulations is essential for maintaining the trust of patients and ensuring the responsible and ethical use of digital health data [58].

Telemedicine, like any other form of electronic communication, is subjected to data security issues such as hacking, data breaches, and unauthorized access to patient information. To protect patient data, telemedicine providers should use secure communication methods, such as encrypted messaging and video conferencing, and comply with relevant regulations. Additionally, providers should regularly update their security measures and train staff on best practices for protecting patient data [61]. Telemedicine is a rapidly growing field with a lot of promise for improving healthcare access and outcomes. However, it is crucial for healthcare professionals to play a central role in ensuring that telemedicine visits are conducted properly and that the technology used respects patient privacy and provides high-quality care [62]. To achieve this, a comprehensive security monitoring policy is necessary. This policy should not only identify vulnerable and suspicious code but also encourage developers to adopt strong defenses against potential hacking and cloning activities [33].

At the same time, it is important for providers to use native digital health software and apps, as they are more likely to meet regulatory requirements and be more secure. Unfortunately, the most commonly used apps, such as WhatsApp, Skype, and Zoom, do not fully comply with telemedicine requirements, as reported by various studies. This highlights the need for more robust and secure telemedicine solutions [63–68].

A study that was performed for over 20,000 health-related smartphone apps, found that a significant number of these apps could potentially access and share personal information, such as email addresses and geolocation data. This raises serious privacy concerns and highlights the need for more stringent data protection policies and security measures. In conclusion, while telemedicine has the potential to transform healthcare, it is important to address these security and privacy concerns to ensure that telemedicine is used in a responsible and effective manner [46].

Despite the benefits of using HIPAA and GDPR-compliant apps and software, their adoption remains limited [69]. To fully realize the potential of digital health and to advance global health goals, such as universal health coverage, a comprehensive data management framework that addresses the needs of real populations must be established at the national and international levels. Additionally, the advancement of international interoperability standards will improve the monitoring of health needs and the delivery of effective interventions [33].

Governments have a key role to play in enabling digital health innovation and addressing the privacy, accountability, and security of health data [70].

Similarly, another great concern is that of legacy liabilities. Telemedicine providers can be held liable for any medical errors or omissions that occur during virtual consultations, and it is important to ensure that they have the appropriate level of training and expertise, follow the same standards of care as in-person consultations, and have malpractice insurance [50,69]. According to Solimini et al., the use of telemedicine should also complement traditional healthcare services rather than replace them [62].

It is important to note that laws and regulations regarding telemedicine may vary by country, and it is important to be aware of the specific laws and regulations that apply in your jurisdiction. In addition, telemedicine raises important questions regarding ethical and legal issues, such as patient privacy and the security of health data, that must be addressed [44]. While telemedicine appears to provide many benefits, such as increased access to care and improved patient convenience, it is critical to address the security, ethical, and legal challenges that come with it as soon as possible in order to fully realize its potential and ensure its safe and effective implementation.

Limitations

This review has limitations, such as the exclusion of non-English articles, limited search sources (PubMed and Scopus), and no search sources for gray area literature.

By only focusing on articles that deal with digital health regulation, particularly data security, privacy, and legacy issues, the study may overlook other important aspects of the topic and may not provide a comprehensive view of the field. This narrow focus could also result in a skewed representation of the current state of research in this area.

5. Conclusions

Digital health has revolutionized the way medical services are delivered. The use of technology has made it possible for patients to receive advice and treatment remotely, ensuring their safety, especially during the COVID-19 pandemic. This has improved access to healthcare for people who may have difficulty traveling to see a doctor in person.

However, the digital health industry faces several challenges. One of the main challenges is the lack of standardized protocols for handling sensitive patient data that apply globally. This raises concerns about the confidentiality and security of patient information, especially in an era where data privacy is a major issue. Additionally, the absence of common legislative provisions regarding the exchange of confidential data makes it difficult to ensure that the delivery of effective care is maintained across different countries and regions.

To address these challenges, regulatory compliance is crucial. It will help clarify and harmonize all regulatory and normative aspects affecting digital health, making it possible to implement these services and make telemedicine mainstream. This will not only improve patient outcomes but also provide doctors with more certainty in their work, as they will know that they are following guidelines that have been established and agreed upon by regulatory authorities.

Another important consideration in the digital health landscape is the emergence of the informed "patient 4.0". This patient is often very well-informed about their health status and is not afraid to ask specific questions and challenge doctors, like a true expert. This can sometimes lead to defensive medicine, in which doctors, out of fear of making mistakes, could prescribe unnecessary tests and procedures. In an unregulated field such as digital health, this could be a major problem, and it is important to address it.

In conclusion, as a result of this scoping review, the authors determined that digital health has improved access to medical services. However, there are still major challenges that need to be addressed. Regulating the handling of patient data, clarifying legislative provisions, and addressing the challenges posed by informed patients are all critical steps in ensuring the successful implementation of telemedicine.

Author Contributions: Conceptualization, O.D.F. and G.L.M.; methodology, M.G.C.A.C. and G.L.M.; validation, G.C.; formal analysis, G.L.M.; investigation and data curation, O.D.F. and G.L.M.; writing—original draft preparation, O.D.F., M.G.C.A.C. and G.L.M.; writing—review and editing, O.D.F. and G.C.; supervision and project administration, G.C. All authors have read and agreed to the published version of the manuscript.

Funding: This research received no funding.

Institutional Review Board Statement: Not applicable.

Informed Consent Statement: Not applicable.

Data Availability Statement: Not applicable.

Conflicts of Interest: The authors declare that there is no conflict of interest.

References

1. Ali, S.A.; El Ansari, W. Is Tele-Diagnosis of Dental Conditions Reliable during COVID-19 Pandemic? Agreement between Tentative Diagnosis via Synchronous Audioconferencing and Definitive Clinical Diagnosis. *J. Dent.* **2022**, *122*, 104144. [CrossRef]
2. Gurgel-Juarez, N.; Torres-Pereira, C.; Haddad, A.E.; Sheehy, L.; Finestone, H.; Mallet, K.; Wiseman, M.; Hour, K.; Flowers, H.L. Accuracy and Effectiveness of Teledentistry: A Systematic Review of Systematic Reviews. *Evid. Based Dent.* **2022**, *23*, 1–8. [CrossRef]
3. Ghai, S. Teledentistry during COVID-19 Pandemic. *Diabetes Metab. Syndr.* **2020**, *14*, 933–935. [CrossRef] [PubMed]
4. Turkistani, K.A. Precautions and Recommendations for Orthodontic Settings during the COVID-19 Outbreak: A Review. *Am. J. Orthod. Dentofac. Orthop.* **2020**, *158*, 175–181. [CrossRef]
5. Nejatidanesh, F.; Khosravi, Z.; Goroohi, H.; Badrian, H.; Savabi, O. Risk of Contamination of Different Areas of Dentist's Face during Dental Practices. *Int. J. Prev. Med.* **2013**, *4*, 611. [PubMed]
6. Peng, X.; Xu, X.; Li, Y.; Cheng, L.; Zhou, X.; Ren, B. Transmission Routes of 2019-NCoV and Controls in Dental Practice. *Int. J. Oral Sci.* **2020**, *12*, 611–615. [CrossRef]
7. Almubarak, H. The Potential Role of Telemedicine in Early Detection of Oral Cancer: A Literature Review. *J. Pharm. Bioallied Sci.* **2022**, *14*, 19. [CrossRef] [PubMed]
8. Jampani, N.D.; Nutalapati, R.; Dontula, B.S.K.; Boyapati, R. Applications of Teledentistry: A Literature Review and Update. *J. Int. Soc. Prev. Community Dent.* **2011**, *1*, 37–44. [CrossRef]
9. Catan, G.; Espanha, R.; Mendes, R.V.; Toren, O.; Chinitz, D. Health Information Technology Implementation-Impacts and Policy Considerations: A Comparison between Israel and Portugal. *Isr. J. Health Policy Res.* **2015**, *4*, 41. [CrossRef]
10. Moen, A.; Hackl, W.O.; Hofdijk, J.; Van Gemert-Pijnen, L.; Ammenwerth, E.; Nykänen, P.; Hoerbst, A. EHealth in Europe-Status and Challenges. *Yearb. Med. Inform.* **2013**, *8*, 59–63. [CrossRef]
11. Callens, S. *The EU Legal Framework on E-Health. Health Systems Governance in Europe: The Role of European Union Law and Policy*; Cambridge University Press: Cambridge, UK, 2010; pp. 561–588. [CrossRef]
12. Lewis, J.; Ray, P.; Liaw, S.T. Recent Worldwide Developments in EHealth and MHealth to More Effectively Manage Cancer and Other Chronic Diseases–A Systematic Review. *Yearb. Med. Inform.* **2016**, *25*, 93–108. [CrossRef]
13. Haleem, A.; Javaid, M.; Singh, R.P.; Suman, R. Telemedicine for Healthcare: Capabilities, Features, Barriers, and Applications. *Sens. Int.* **2021**, *2*, 100117. [CrossRef]
14. Terry, M. Telemedicine and E-Health. 2010. Available online: https://home.liebertpub.com/tmj (accessed on 13 March 2023).
15. Maaß, L.; Freye, M.; Pan, C.C.; Dassow, H.H.; Niess, J.; Jahnel, T. The Definitions of Health Apps and Medical Apps from the Perspective of Public Health and Law: Qualitative Analysis of an Interdisciplinary Literature Overview. *JMIR Mhealth Uhealth* **2022**, *10*, e37980. [CrossRef]

16. Digital in 2019: Global Internet Use Accelerates-We Are Social UK. Available online: https://wearesocial.com/uk/blog/2019/01/digital-in-2019-global-internet-use-accelerates/ (accessed on 7 March 2023).
17. Thomas, K. Wanted: A WhatsApp Alternative for Clinicians. *BMJ* **2018**, *360*, k622. [CrossRef]
18. Giansanti, D. WhatsApp in MHealth: An Overview on the Potentialities and the Opportunities in Medical Imaging. *Mhealth* **2020**, *6*, 19. [CrossRef]
19. Koparal, M.; Ünsal, H.Y.; Alan, H.; Üçkardeş, F.; Gülsün, B. WhatsApp Messaging Improves Communication in an Oral and Maxillofacial Surgery Team. *Int. J. Med. Inform.* **2019**, *132*, 103987. [CrossRef]
20. Mohamed, I.N.; Elseed, M.A. Utility of WhatsApp in Healthcare Provision and Sharing of Medical Information with Caregivers of Children with Neurodisabilties: Experience from Sudan. *Sudan. J. Paediatr.* **2021**, *21*, 48. [CrossRef]
21. Salam, M.A.U.; Oyekwe, G.C.; Ghani, S.A.; Choudhury, R.I. How Can WhatsApp® Facilitate the Future of Medical Education and Clinical Practice? *BMC Med. Educ.* **2021**, *21*, 54. [CrossRef]
22. Mars, M.; Escott, R. WhatsApp in Clinical Practice: A Literature Review. *Stud. Health Technol. Inform.* **2016**, *231*, 82–90. [CrossRef]
23. Masoni, M.; Guelfi, M.R. WhatsApp and Other Messaging Apps in Medicine: Opportunities and Risks. *Intern. Emerg. Med.* **2020**, *15*, 171–173. [CrossRef]
24. Mars, M.; Morris, C.; Scott, R.E. WhatsApp Guidelines-What Guidelines? A Literature Review. *J. Telemed. Telecare* **2019**, *25*, 524–529. [CrossRef]
25. Mahmoud, K.; Jaramillo, C.; Barteit, S. Telemedicine in Low- and Middle-Income Countries During the COVID-19 Pandemic: A Scoping Review. *Front. Public Health* **2022**, *10*, 1854. [CrossRef]
26. Lee Ventola, C. Social Media and Health Care Professionals: Benefits, Risks, and Best Practices. *Pharm. Ther.* **2014**, *39*, 491.
27. Wani, S.A.; Rabah, S.M.; Alfadil, S.; Dewanjee, N.; Najmi, Y. Efficacy of Communication amongst Staff Members at Plastic and Reconstructive Surgery Section Using Smartphone and Mobile WhatsApp. *Indian J. Plast. Surg.* **2013**, *46*, 502. [CrossRef]
28. Khanna, V.; Sambandam, S.N.; Gul, A.; Mounasamy, V. "WhatsApp" Ening in Orthopedic Care: A Concise Report from a 300-Bedded Tertiary Care Teaching Center. *Eur. J. Orthop. Surg. Traumatol.* **2015**, *25*, 821–826. [CrossRef]
29. Choudhari, P. Study on Effectiveness of Communication amongst Members at Department of Orthopedics Surgery Unit 3 Using Smartphone and Mobile WhatsApp. *Int. Surg. J.* **2016**, *1*, 9–12. [CrossRef]
30. The Use of Smartphones or Tablets in Surgery. What Are the Limits?—Annali Italiani Di Chirurgia. Available online: https://www.annaliitalianidichirurgia.it/prodotto/the-use-of-smartphones-or-tablets-in-surgery-what-are-the-limits/ (accessed on 8 March 2023).
31. Dhuvad, J.M.; Dhuvad, M.M.; Kshirsagar, R.A. Have Smartphones Contributed in the Clinical Progress of Oral and Maxillofacial Surgery? *J. Clin. Diagn. Res.* **2015**, *9*, ZC22–ZC24. [CrossRef]
32. Senthoor Pandian, S.; Srinivasan, P.; Mohan, S. The Maxillofacial Surgeon's March towards a Smarter Future-Smartphones. *J. Maxillofac. Oral Surg.* **2014**, *13*, 355–358. [CrossRef]
33. Parker, L.; Karliychuk, T.; Gillies, D.; Mintzes, B.; Raven, M.; Grundy, Q. A Health App Developer's Guide to Law and Policy: A Multi-Sector Policy Analysis. *BMC Med. Inform. Decis. Mak.* **2017**, *17*, 141. [CrossRef]
34. Liu, X.; Sutton, P.R.; McKenna, R.; Sinanan, M.N.; Fellner, B.J.; Leu, M.G.; Ewell, C. Evaluation of Secure Messaging Applications for a Health Care System: A Case Study. *Appl. Clin. Inform.* **2019**, *10*, 140–150. [CrossRef]
35. Agarwal, N.; Jain, P.; Pathak, R.; Gupta, R. Telemedicine in India: A Tool for Transforming Health Care in the Era of COVID-19 Pandemic. *J. Educ. Heal. Promot.* **2020**, *9*, 190. [CrossRef]
36. Benjumea, J.; Ropero, J.; Rivera-Romero, O.; Dorronzoro-Zubiete, E.; Carrasco, A. Privacy Assessment in Mobile Health Apps: Scoping Review. *JMIR Mhealth Uhealth* **2020**, *8*, e18868. [CrossRef]
37. Caetano, R.; Silva, A.B.; Guedes, A.C.C.M.; de Paiva, C.C.N.; da Rocha Ribeiro, G.; Santos, D.L.; da Silva, R.M. Challenges and Opportunities for Telehealth during the COVID-19 Pandemic: Ideas on Spaces and Initiatives in the Brazilian Context. *Cad. Saude Publica* **2020**, *36*, e00088920. [CrossRef]
38. Ghosh, A.; Gupta, R.; Misra, A. Telemedicine for Diabetes Care in India during COVID-19 Pandemic and National Lockdown Period: Guidelines for Physicians. *Diabetes Metab. Syndr.* **2020**, *14*, 273–276. [CrossRef]
39. Kaplan, B. Revisiting health information technology ethical, legal, and social issues and evaluation: Telehealth/telemedicine and COVID-19. *Int. J. Med. Inform.* **2020**, *143*, 104239. [CrossRef]
40. Mahtta, D.; Daher, M.; Lee, M.T.; Sayani, S.; Shishehbor, M.; Virani, S.S. Promise and Perils of Telehealth in the Current Era. *Curr. Cardiol. Rep.* **2021**, *23*, 115. [CrossRef]
41. Kichloo, A.; Albosta, M.; Dettloff, K.; Wani, F.; El-Amir, Z.; Singh, J.; Aljadah, M.; Chakinala, R.C.; Kanugula, A.K.; Solanki, S.; et al. Telemedicine, the Current COVID-19 Pandemic and the Future: A Narrative Review and Perspectives Moving Forward in the USA. *Fam. Med. Community Health* **2020**, *8*, e000530. [CrossRef]
42. Moura, P.; Fazendeiro, P.; Inácio, P.R.M.; Vieira-Marques, P.; Ferreira, A. Assessing Access Control Risk for MHealth: A Delphi Study to Categorize Security of Health Data and Provide Risk Assessment for Mobile Apps. *J. Healthc. Eng.* **2020**, *2020*, 5601068. [CrossRef]
43. Gowda, V.; Cheng, G.; Harvey, H.B. Safeguarding Data Security in the Era of Imaging MHealth. *AJR Am. J. Roentgenol.* **2021**, *218*, 820–821. [CrossRef]
44. Hoaglin, M.C.; Brenner, L.H.; Teo, W.; Bal, B.S. Medicolegal Sidebar: Telemedicine-New Opportunities and New Risks. *Clin. Orthop. Relat. Res.* **2021**, *479*, 1671–1673. [CrossRef]

45. Pool, J.; Akhlaghpour, S.; Fatehi, F. Health Data Privacy in the COVID-19 Pandemic Context: Discourses on HIPAA. *Stud. Health Technol. Inform.* **2021**, *279*, 70–77. [CrossRef]
46. Tangari, G.; Ikram, M.; Ijaz, K.; Kaafar, M.A.; Berkovsky, S. Mobile Health and Privacy: Cross Sectional Study. *BMJ* **2021**, *373*, n1248. [CrossRef] [PubMed]
47. Alfawzan, N.; Christen, M.; Spitale, G.; Biller-Andorno, N. Privacy, Data Sharing, and Data Security Policies of Women's MHealth Apps: Scoping Review and Content Analysis. *JMIR Mhealth Uhealth* **2022**, *10*, e33735. [CrossRef] [PubMed]
48. Essén, A.; Stern, A.D.; Haase, C.B.; Car, J.; Greaves, F.; Paparova, D.; Vandeput, S.; Wehrens, R.; Bates, D.W. Health App Policy: International Comparison of Nine Countries' Approaches. *NPJ Digit. Med.* **2022**, *5*, 31. [CrossRef]
49. Grundy, Q. A Review of the Quality and Impact of Mobile Health Apps. *Annu. Rev. Public Health* **2022**, *43*, 117–134. [CrossRef] [PubMed]
50. Mazzuca, D.; Borselli, M.; Gratteri, S.; Zampogna, G.; Feola, A.; Della Corte, M.; Guarna, F.; Scorcia, V.; Giannaccare, G. Applications and Current Medico-Legal Challenges of Telemedicine in Ophthalmology. *J. Environ. Res. Public Health* **2022**, *19*, 5614. [CrossRef]
51. Sujarwoto, S.; Augia, T.; Dahlan, H.; Sahputri, R.A.M.; Holipah, H.; Maharani, A. COVID-19 Mobile Health Apps: An Overview of Mobile Applications in Indonesia. *Front. Public Health* **2022**, *10*, 879695. [CrossRef]
52. Venkatesh, U.; Aravind, G.P.; Velmurugan, A.A. Telemedicine Practice Guidelines in India: Global Implications in the Wake of the COVID-19 Pandemic. *World Med. Health Policy* **2022**, *14*, 589–599. [CrossRef]
53. Eisenstein, E.; Kopacek, C.; Cavalcante, S.S.; Neves, A.C.; Fraga, G.P.; Messina, L.A. Telemedicine: A Bridge Over Knowledge Gaps in Healthcare. *Curr. Pediatr. Rep.* **2020**, *8*, 93–98. [CrossRef]
54. Perez-Noboa, B.; Soledispa-Carrasco, A.; Sanchez Padilla, V.; Velasquez, W. Teleconsultation Apps in the COVID-19 Pandemic: The Case of Guayaquil City, Ecuador. *IEEE Eng. Manag. Rev.* **2021**, *49*, 27–37. [CrossRef]
55. Wang, C.J.; Liu, T.T.; Car, J.; Zuckerman, B. Design, Adoption, Implementation, Scalability, and Sustainability of Telehealth Programs. *Pediatr. Clin. N. Am.* **2020**, *67*, 675–682. [CrossRef]
56. Lee, D.W.H.; Tong, K.W.; Lai, P.B.S. Telehealth Practice in Surgery: Ethical and Medico-legal Considerations. *Surg. Pract.* **2021**, *25*, 42. [CrossRef]
57. Ferorelli, D.; Moretti, L.; Benevento, M.; Mastrapasqua, M.; Telegrafo, M.; Solarino, B.; Dell'Erba, A.; Bizzoca, D.; Moretti, B. Digital Health Care, Telemedicine, and Medicolegal Issues in Orthopedics: A Review. *Int. J. Environ. Res. Public Health* **2022**, *19*, 15653. [CrossRef] [PubMed]
58. Tangari, G.; Ikram, M.; Sentana, I.W.B.; Ijaz, K.; Kaafar, M.A.; Berkovsky, S. Analyzing Security Issues of Android Mobile Health and Medical Applications. *J. Am. Med. Inform. Assoc.* **2021**, *28*, 2074. [CrossRef] [PubMed]
59. Hussein, R.; Wurhofer, D.; Strumegger, E.M.; Stainer-Hochgatterer, A.; Kulnik, S.T.; Crutzen, R.; Niebauer, J. General Data Protection Regulation (GDPR) Toolkit for Digital Health. *Stud. Health Technol. Inform.* **2022**, *290*, 222–226. [CrossRef]
60. Kruse, C.S.; Smith, B.; Vanderlinden, H.; Nealand, A. Security Techniques for the Electronic Health Records. *J. Med Syst.* **2017**, *41*, 127. [CrossRef] [PubMed]
61. Schütze, D.; Engler, F.; Nohl-Deryk, P.; Müller, B.; Müller, A. Implementing a Secure Instant Messaging App in the COVID-19 Pandemic: Usage Experiences of Primary Care Physicians and Local Health Authorities. *Z. Evid. Fortbild. Qual. Gesundhwes.* **2022**, *173*, 40–48. [CrossRef] [PubMed]
62. Solimini, R.; Busardò, F.P.; Gibelli, F.; Sirignano, A.; Ricci, G. Ethical and Legal Challenges of Telemedicine in the Era of the COVID-19 Pandemic. *Medicina* **2021**, *57*, 1314. [CrossRef]
63. Chung, K.; Wong, J.; Cunha-Cruz, J.; Carsten, D. Teledentistry: An Adjunct for Delivering Dental Care in Crises and Beyond. *Compend. Contin. Educ. Dent.* **2022**, *43*, 108–112.
64. Alsafwani, Z.; Shiboski, C.; Villa, A. The Role of Telemedicine for Symptoms Management in Oral Medicine: A Retrospective Observational Study. *BMC Oral Health* **2022**, *22*, 92. [CrossRef]
65. Patel, T.; Wong, J. The Role of Real-Time Interactive Video Consultations in Dental Practice during the Recovery and Restoration Phase of the COVID-19 Outbreak. *Br. Dent. J.* **2020**, *229*, 196–200. [CrossRef]
66. Wu, D.T.; Wu, K.Y.; Nguyen, T.T.; Tran, S.D. The Impact of COVID-19 on Dental Education in North America-Where Do We Go Next? *Eur. J. Dent. Educ.* **2020**, *24*, 825–827. [CrossRef]
67. Farooq, I.; Ali, S.; Alam Moheet, I.; Alhumaid, J. COVID-19 Outbreak, Disruption of Dental Education, and the Role of Teledentistry. *Pak. J. Med. Sci.* **2020**, *36*, 1726. [CrossRef]
68. Doraiswamy, S.; Abraham, A.; Mamtani, R.; Cheema, S. Use of Telehealth during the COVID-19 Pandemic: Scoping Review. *J. Med. Internet Res.* **2020**, *22*, e24087. [CrossRef] [PubMed]
69. Oliva, A.; Grassi, S.; Vetrugno, G.; Rossi, R.; Della Morte, G.; Pinchi, V.; Caputo, M. Management of Medico-Legal Risks in Digital Health Era: A Scoping Review. *Front. Med.* **2022**, *8*, 2956. [CrossRef] [PubMed]
70. Wong, B.L.H.; Maaß, L.; Vodden, A.; van Kessel, R.; Sorbello, S.; Buttigieg, S.; Odone, A. The Dawn of Digital Public Health in Europe: Implications for Public Health Policy and Practice. *Lancet Reg. Health Eur.* **2022**, *14*, 100316. [CrossRef] [PubMed]

Disclaimer/Publisher's Note: The statements, opinions and data contained in all publications are solely those of the individual author(s) and contributor(s) and not of MDPI and/or the editor(s). MDPI and/or the editor(s) disclaim responsibility for any injury to people or property resulting from any ideas, methods, instructions or products referred to in the content.

Review

Photodynamic Therapy of Oral Cancer and Novel Liposomal Photosensitizers [†]

Nejat Düzgüneş [1,*], Jaroslaw Piskorz [2], Paulina Skupin-Mrugalska [2], Metin Yıldırım [3], Melike Sessevmez [4] and Jennifer Cheung [1]

[1] Department of Biomedical Sciences, Arthur A. Dugoni School of Dentistry, University of the Pacific, 155 Fifth Street, San Francisco, CA 94103, USA; jgcheung@ucla.edu
[2] Department of Inorganic and Analytical Chemistry, Poznan University of Medical Sciences, Rokietnicka 3, 60-806 Poznan, Poland; piskorzj@ump.edu.pl (J.P.); p_skupin@wp.pl (P.S.-M.)
[3] Department of Pharmacy Services, Vocational School of Health Services, Tarsus University, Mersin 33400, Turkey; metinyildirim4@gmail.com
[4] Department of Pharmaceutical Technology, Faculty of Pharmacy, Istanbul University, Istanbul 34452, Turkey; melikesessevmez@gmail.com
* Correspondence: nduzgunes@pacific.edu
[†] This paper is dedicated to the memory of Krystyna Konopka, formerly Professor of Microbiology and of Biomedical Sciences at the Arthur A. Dugoni School of Dentistry.

Abstract: Photodynamic therapy facilitates the selective destruction of cancer tissue by utilizing a photosensitizer drug, the light near the absorbance wavelength of the drug, and oxygen. Methylene Blue, 5-aminolevulinic acid (the precursor of the photosensitizer, protoporphyrin IX), porphyrin, Foscan, Chlorin e6, and HPPH have been used successfully as photosensitizers in the treatment of oral verrucous hyperplasia, oral leukoplakia, oral lichen planus, and head and neck squamous cell carcinoma. "Theranostic" liposomes can deliver a contrast agent for magnetic resonance imaging and a photosensitizer for the image-guided photodynamic therapy of head and neck cancer. Liposomes incorporating photosensitizers can be targeted to cell surface markers overexpressed on cancer cells. Novel porphyrinoids have been developed in our laboratories that are highly effective as photosensitizers. Tribenzoporphyrazines encapsulated in cationic liposomes have produced IC_{50} values up to 50 times lower compared to the free photosensitizers. It is anticipated that targeting these drugs to cancer stem cells, using upconversion nanoparticles for the near-infrared irradiation of tumors to activate the photosensitizers, and overcoming tumor hypoxia will enhance the efficacy of photodynamic therapy of tumors accessible to light sources.

Keywords: oral squamous cell carcinoma; pharyngeal cancer; nanoparticles; photodynamic therapy; photosensitizer; targeted liposomes; singlet excited state; theranostics; tribenzoporphyrazines

1. Introduction

The World Cancer Research Fund International reports that, in 2020, the incidence of mouth and oral cancer was 744,994 throughout the world. The number of deaths during this period was 364,339 [1]. The Oral Cancer Foundation estimates that the worldwide burden of cancers of the oral cavity and oropharynx is 657,000 new cases per year, and more than 330,000 deaths.

Of the newly diagnosed persons, only slightly more than half will be alive within 5 years. This outcome has not changed significantly over several decades, except in the case of HPV16-positive oral cancers that respond better to current treatments. Surgery generally leads to disfiguration. Chemotherapy and radiation therapy cause difficulty in swallowing, chewing and talking, jaw pain, mouth sores, and dysfunctional salivary glands.

Photodynamic therapy makes possible the selective destruction of cancer tissue, and may complement surgery, radiotherapy and chemotherapy. Photodynamic therapy utilizes a photosensitizer drug, the light at or near the absorbance wavelength of the drug, and oxygen. The incidence of light on the photosensitizer, which is initially in the low energy ground "singlet state" (S_0) and has two electrons with opposite spins (corresponding to a total spin angular momentum of *zero*), generates the "singlet-excited state" (S_1 or S_2) with the electrons in an orbital with a higher energy (Figure 1) [2]. The singlet excited-state is not stable and loses its energy by alternate mechanisms: (i) emitting light, observed as fluorescence at a higher wavelength (i.e., lower energy; the Stokes shift); (ii) heat production via a process termed "internal conversion"; or (iii) "intersystem crossing", forming the excited "triplet state" with a total spin angular momentum of *one*, arising from parallel spinning electrons. The triplet simply means that, in this state, the molecule exhibits three spectral lines of light absorption.

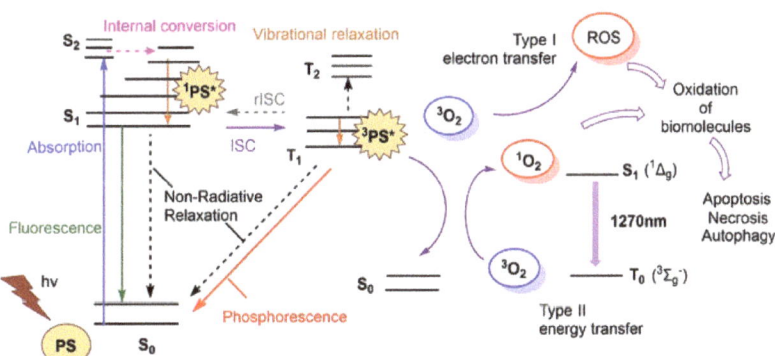

Figure 1. Simplified Jablonski diagram, showing the pathways after photoactivation of a photosensitizer (PS). When the photosensitizer absorbs light (with an energy given by $h\nu$, where h is Planck's constant, and ν is the frequency of light) an electron in the singlet ground state is energized into a high-energy singlet state. This state can lose energy by emitting a photon at a higher wavelength (fluorescence) or by internal conversion (non-radiative relaxation). The spin of the high-energy electron may flip in intersystem crossing (ISC), forming the excited triplet state, which has a relatively long half-life. Superoxide and hydroxyl radicals are formed in the presence of molecular oxygen in Type I reactions. Singlet oxygen is formed in Type II reactions. These reactive oxygen species can damage amino acids, lipids and nucleic acids (Reproduced with permission from Melissari et al. [3]).

In the ensuing "Type I" reaction, the photosensitizer in the triplet state can interact with a neighboring molecule, which may be an electron donor or electron acceptor, forming a radical anion or a radical cation, which can then react with oxygen to form the superoxide radical ($O_2^-\bullet$), hydrogen peroxide (H_2O_2), and hydroxyl radicals ($HO\bullet$) (Figure 1). In the "Type II" reaction, the energy of the triplet state photosensitizer is transferred to ground state triplet molecular oxygen (O_2), producing the highly reactive excited singlet oxygen ($^1O_2$) (Figure 1). These reactive oxygen species (ROS) can then oxidize proteins, nucleic acids and lipids, resulting in cytotoxicity to a cancer cell or a microorganism. Photosensitizers employed in cancer treatment mostly utilize the Type II mechanism [2].

An oxygen-independent mechanism of photodynamic therapy, termed Type III, has been described whereby excited photosensitizers directly degrade nucleic acids and proteins [4,5].

Photodynamic therapy can cause an increase in the intracellular Ca^{2+} concentration and the activation of phospholipase A_2 [6]. It can down-regulate the epidermal growth factor receptor at the cell surface. It can cause the accumulation of ceramide, leading to an increase in mitochondrial membrane permeability and the release of cytochrome c. Photodynamic therapy can result in the expression of interleukin-6 and integrin damage.

The anti-cancer effect by photodynamic therapy may be caused by (i) direct cytotoxicity to cancer cells, (ii) occlusion of the tumor vasculature, thus causing hypoxia and cell death, or (iii) induction of a systemic immune response directed at the tumor [6]. Cytotoxicity may be mediated by apoptosis, necrosis, and possibly autophagy. For example, photodynamic therapy with 5-aminolevulinic acid induces apoptosis in the oral cancer cell line, CA9-22, via the NF-kB/JNK pathway, and involves both caspase 8-and caspase-9 [7]. Pheophorbide a is a photosensitizer that was synthesized by the removal of a magnesium ion and a phytyl group from chlorophyll-a [8]. Photodynamic therapy in human oral squamous cell carcinoma cells, YD-10B, utilizing pheophorbide a, inhibits the proliferation of the cells, increases the number of apoptotic cells via the inactivation of the ERK pathway, and also induces autophagy, shown by the increased expression of microtubule-associated protein 1 light chain 3B and the accumulation of acidic vesicular organelles [8]. Another important mechanism that contributes to photodynamic therapy therapeutic performance involves the activation of the immunological system. Thus, at some point, photodynamic therapy can be considered as a cancer immunotherapy. Treatment with various classes of photosensitizers is known to trigger immunogenic cell death (ICD) where the T-cell adaptive immune response is activated, leading to the formation of long-term immunological memory [5,9].

A major advantage of photodynamic therapy over conventional treatments is its minimal invasiveness, as well as relatively selective tumor destruction and the preservation of healthy tissues [10]. Some photosensitizers can concentrate in tumors relative to the surrounding healthy tissue [11–13]. Liposomes targeted to the transferrin receptor can mediate an 18-fold higher accumulation of the photosensitizer, aluminum phthalocyanine tetrasulfonate, in bladder tumors compared to normal urothelium [14]. These properties are significant in the treatment of head and neck squamous cell carcinoma, where loss of normal tissue may cause functional problems and disfiguration. Photodynamic therapy may also be used in combination with conventional treatments [15].

Below, we discuss the use of various photosensitizers in the treatment of head and neck squamous cell carcinoma in patients, in animal models, and in vitro, as well as describe the novel photosensitizers developed in our laboratories.

2. 5-Aminolevulinic Acid

The compound 5-aminolevulinic acid is a precursor of the photosensitizer, protoporphyrin IX, in the heme biosynthetic pathway [10,16]. Exogenous 5-aminolevulinic acid (Figure 2) inhibits the first step of porphyrin synthesis, which thus results in the accumulation of protoporphyrin IX in the tissue.

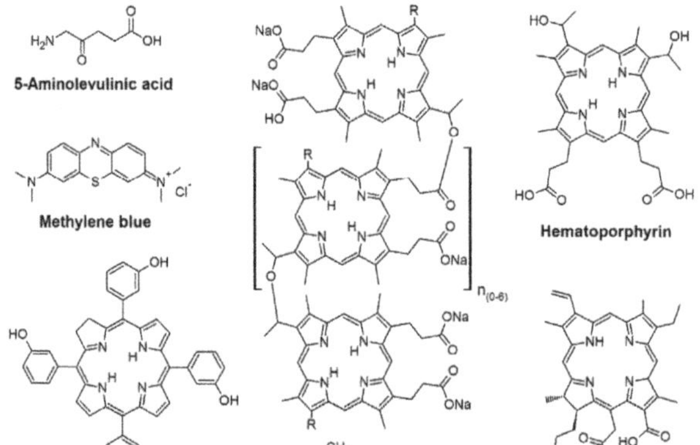

Figure 2. Molecular structures of photosensitizers.

Photodynamic therapy with 5-aminolevulinic acid has been used fairly widely in clinical studies against oral leukoplakia, which has the potential to become malignant [17]. Correspondingly, oral leukoplakia presents a convenient clinical model for cancer preventive approaches [18]. One of the earlier attempts to treat oral leukoplakia with 5-aminolevulinic acid was that of Kübler et al. [19], which involved the application of a 20% 5-aminolevulinic acid cream, locally for 2 h, to 12 patients who had had oral leukoplakia for many years. After removing the cream, monochromatic red light at 630 nm from an argon-dye laser (at a radiant exposure of 100 J/cm^2) was applied to the leukoplakia lesions of the patients for 1 h. After 3 months of therapy, five patients were cured completely.

Four patients showed a partial response, while three patients did not show any response [19]. Similar to this study, Sieron et al. [20] reported that a complete response was achieved in 10 out of 12 patients suffering from oral leukoplakia when they were treated with a 10% 5-aminolevulinic acid emulsion (O/W) topically with 6–8 irradiation sessions utilizing an Argon-pumped dye laser at 635 nm (delivering a total dose of 100 J/cm^2 per session). To examine treatment efficacy in different diseases and treatment protocols, Chen et al. [21] topically applied a 20% 5-aminolevulinic acid gel to 32 patients, including 8 patients with oral verrucous hyperplasia and 24 patients with oral leukoplakia. Oral verrucous hyperplasia lesions showed a better response than oral leukoplakia lesions to this photodynamic therapy. Oral leukoplakia lesions required the application of the protocol twice a week to show even a partial response, while oral verrucous hyperplasia lesions showed a complete response in fewer than six treatments once a week [21].

Siddiqui et al. [22] reported the effects of photoactivated aminolevulinic acid as an oral cancer therapy. The regimen of the photosensitizing agent is normally 60 mg/kg divided into three doses, which leads to accumulation of the photoactive product protoporphyrin IX (PpIX), followed, after 0.5–1 h, by illumination of the tumor with 100 J/cm^2 LED light at 635 nm. Complete tumor response was achieved in 76% of patients.

Recently, Yao et al. [23] applied an ablative fractional laser to oral leukoplakia lesions in the oral cavity of 48 patients to improve the clinical success of 5-aminolevulinic acid-mediated photodynamic therapy with the aim of enhancing the tissue penetration of the photosensitizer. After this procedure, a 20% gel of 5-aminolevulinic acid was applied topically to the lesions for 3 h, and the areas were illuminated subsequently by red light with a Yage LED-IB at a wavelength of 630 nm (180 J/cm^2). After one month, 30 patients had complete recovery and 12 patients had partial recovery. The recurrence and malignant transformation rates were 37.5% and 8.3%, respectively, after 3 years of follow-up of the patients [23].

3. Methylene Blue

Oral lichen planus is a chronic inflammatory disease that has the risk of transformation into malignant squamous cell carcinoma [24]. The standard treatment for this condition is topically applied corticosteroids that have local side effects, including secondary candidiasis, hypopigmentation, and delayed wound healing, in long-term use [25]. Methylene blue (Figure 2), which has been used as a photosensitizer in the treatment of basal cell carcinoma, Kaposi's sarcoma and melanoma [26], has also been studied for its efficacy and safety in photodynamic therapy for oral lichen planus. Aghahosseini et al. [27] used methylene blue for photodynamic therapy on 13 patients with 26 oral lichen planus lesions. After gargling with a 5% methylene blue solution, laser light was applied to the lesions for 2 min (diode laser, 632 nm, 120 J/cm^2). At the end of 12 weeks of follow-up, 16 of the lesions showed significant reduction in size, with an average reduction of around 44%. In addition, no serious side effects were observed in the patients [27]. In a similar study, 20 patients with oral lichen planus underwent methylene blue-mediated photodynamic therapy. Four weeks after the treatment, 17 of 20 patients responded to treatment. Three patients did not respond to treatment because of longer-term lesions and because the implied duration of the lesion may be a determinant in the response to treatment [28].

Bakhtiari et al. [29] compared the efficacy of methylene-blue-mediated photodynamic therapy with conventional topical corticosteroid treatment on 30 patients with oral lichen planus. After 60 days of follow up, photodynamic therapy was found to be as effective as corticosteroid therapy and had no side effects [29]. Mostafa et al. [30], however, reported that methylene-blue-mediated photodynamic therapy (diode laser, wavelength 660 nm, intensity 100–130 mW/cm^2) gave better results in terms of size reduction in the lesions and of pain compared to topical corticosteroid treatment. These clinical trials indicate that photodynamic therapy with methylene blue has the potential to be used as an alternative to conventional corticosteroid therapy [30].

4. Porphyrin Photosensitizers

Photofrin (dihematoporphyrin ether) and hematoporphyrin derivatives are referred to as first-generation sensitizers [10] (Figure 2). Biel has studied the treatment of a large group of head and neck squamous cell carcinoma patients with Photofrin. Early on, 'true' cancer of the larynx was treated successfully. A complete response was observed in about 90% of patients, even in those who failed an initial therapy (usually radiation) [15,31–33]. Biel [33] reported the use of Photofrin photodynamic therapy on 110 patients with recurrent or primary laryngeal tumors. The therapy involved the intravenous injection of 2 mg/kg photosensitizer, and treatment 48 h later with light from an Nd:Yag pumped-dye laser (Laserscope) at 630 nm, using a 400-mm fused silica optical fiber (Laserguide) and a microlens. The light dose rate was 80 J/cm^2 and 150 mW/cm^2 in the larynx. A 5-year cure rate of 90% was achieved, and all the recurrences could be treated with photodynamic therapy, surgery or radiation.

Biel [33] has suggested that photodynamic therapy should be considered for the treatment of primary and recurrent Tis (in situ carcinoma in the superficial lining of the oral cavity), T1 (tumor $\leq$ 2 cm across), and T2 (tumor > 2 cm and <4 cm across) squamous cell carcinoma of the larynx.

Porfimer sodium (Photofrin)-mediated photodynamic therapy was employed to treat 18 patients with squamous cell carcinoma and 7 with epithelial dysplasia with hyperkeratosis in the oral cavity [34]. The patients received intravenous Photofrin at a dose of 2 mg/kg 48 h before laser irradiation. The lesions were irradiated with an excimer dye laser (PDT-EDL1 from Hamamatsu Photonics) at 630 nm, with an irradiation output of 4 mJ/pulse/cm^2, and a repetition rate of 40 Hz. Light was directed to the tumor by means of a 400 µm flat-tipped quartz fiber. Ninety six percent of the patients were cured.

5. Foscan (Temoporfin; mTHPC)

Foscan [5,10,15,20-meta-tetra(hydroxyphenyl)chlorin, Temoporfin, mTHPC] (Figure 2) has been used in the treatment of early oral squamous cell carcinoma in 114 patients who had floor-of-the-mouth, lip, and anterior tongue lesions [35]. Foscan (0.15 mg/kg) was given intravenously and the lesions were exposed to laser light at 652 nm with a total dose of 20 J/cm^2, at a fluence rate of 100 mW/cm^2. The light was delivered to the tumor over 200 s through an optical fiber and microlens diffuser. The response rate was 93% for T1 lesions and 58% for T2 lesions. All patients sustained an excellent functional status after therapy, and none of them required airway management.

D'Cruz et al. [36] reported data on 128 patients with incurable or recurrent disease. Fifteen patients had multiple lesions. Four days after the administration of mTHPC, the tumor surface was illuminated with a nonthermal diode laser using a microlens fiber at a light dose of 20 J/cm^2, and an intensity of 100 mW/cm^2 at 652 nm. Incident light was perpendicular to the tumor surface and illuminated an area 0.5 cm beyond the visible tumor. About 16% of patients achieved a complete response. Thus, it appears that this group of patients, who had already had extensive surgery and radiation, could still benefit from 'salvage' photodynamic therapy [36].

Foscan may also be used in the treatment of lip cancer with better functional outcomes than those achievable by surgery and radiation [37], early oral squamous cell carcinoma [35], as well as advanced head and neck cancer [38].

One hundred and seventy patients, with early-stage (Tis, T1, T2) oral cavity and oropharynx squamous cell cancers or carcinoma in situ, were treated with intravenous Temoporfin at 0.15 mg/kg body weight, followed, after 96 h, by exposure to a diode laser at 652 nm and a dose of 20 J/cm^2. The overall response rate in this study was 91%, with a complete response rate of 71% [39].

Copper et al. performed photodynamic therapy on 25 patients with T1–T2 N0 tumors (tumors that have not spread to the local lymph nodes) of the oral cavity and/or oropharynx. Patients received meta-tetra(hydroxyphenyl) chlorin (mTHPC) (Foscan) as a photosensitizer. The trial resulted in complete remission for 25 patients [40].

In another study, 21 patients with stage IV advanced and/or recurrent tongue base carcinoma were treated with photodynamic therapy using mTHPC (0.15 mg/kg) as a photosensitizer. Fifteen patients did not report problems after the treatment. Photodynamic therapy, in this case, significantly reduced tumor-associated symptoms such as breathing, swallowing, and speech (voice) problems [41].

6. Chlorin e6 and HPPH

Sobaniec et al. studied photodynamic therapy in 23 patients with oral leukoplakia. Patients were treated with chlorin e6 (Photolon®) (Figure 2), containing 20% chlorin e6 and 10% dimethylsulfoxide as a photosensitizer. The appointments were scheduled for PDT treatment biweekly and this treatment reduced the size of the oral leukoplakia lesion [42] by 55% (average).

In a clinical trial involving patients with oral dysplasia, carcinoma in situ, or early-stage head and neck squamous cell carcinoma, patients were given 3-(1′-hexyloxyethyl) pyropheophorbide (HPPH) (Figure 3) at a dose of 4 mg/m^2 systemically, 22–26 h before light delivery. The tumor was illuminated with 50 to 140 J/cm^2. At day 28, there was 58% complete response, 11% partial response, and 11% stable disease [43].

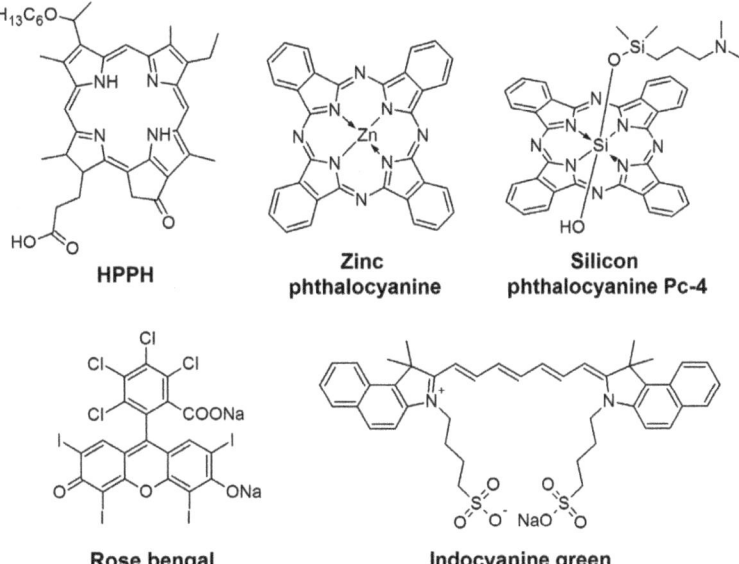

Figure 3. Molecular structure of photosensitizers.

7. Theranostics and Photodynamic Therapy

The theranostic approach relies on combining several modalities, such as imaging, delivery of therapeutics, as well as stimuli-responsive delivery within one system. This strategy is applied to achieve more precise drug delivery, monitor therapy outcomes, enhance tumor penetration, and provide better biocompatibility and more controllable drug release. Sophisticated multifunctional platforms are designed to include all the required modalities.

Theranostic agents have been investigated in the field of photodynamic therapy in various cancer models, with some examples in oral cancer. Recently, we reported on theranostic liposomes delivering a contrast agent (a hybrid of a phospholipid and gadopentetic acid) for magnetic resonance imaging (MRI) and the therapeutic agent, a second-generation photosensitizer, zinc(II) phthalocyanine (ZnPc) (Figure 3). The system has been developed for image-guided photodynamic therapy of head and neck cancer. We observed that, in comparison to liposomes containing only a contrast agent (without ZnPc), the theranostic liposomes (with both Gd(III) chelate and ZnPc) had higher relaxivity. The improved relaxation of theranostic liposomes (resulting from the presence of ZnPc), may possibly enhance MRI contrast, and thus potentially allow a reduction in the Gd(III) chelate dose. The positive influence of ZnPc on relaxivities of theranostic liposomes was attributed to the changes that occur inside the liposomal bilayer that affect water permeability across the liposomal membrane, enabling the interaction of water molecules with paramagnetic centers. Regarding photodynamic efficacy, ZnPc, loaded into theranostic liposomes, exhibit IC_{50} of 0.22–0.61 µM in two oral cancer cellular models (SCC-25 and FaDu) [44].

To reduce the toxicity and improve the performance of photodynamic therapy, targeted platforms for theranostic applications have been developed. Wang et al. [45] studied targeted iron-oxide nanoparticles for photodynamic therapy and MRI of head and neck cancer. The system involved a second-generation photodynamic therapy drug, Pc 4, a cancer-targeting ligand, fibronectin-mimetic peptide (Fmp), and iron oxide nanoparticles. Non-targeted and targeted nanoparticles accumulated in xenograft tumors with higher concentrations than non-formulated Pc 4 and reduced the size of head and neck squamous cell carcinoma xenograft tumors.

Another strategy that allows controllable drug release is the stimuli-responsive drug delivery system [46]. These systems respond to the unique properties of the tumor microenvironment involving acidic pH, the overexpression of specific enzymes, and high levels of ROS. In studies of light-responsive drug delivery systems, a combination of photodynamic therapy and photothermal therapy has been reported, of which the synergistic therapeutic effect was verified [46]. For example, Song et al. [47] designed a chlorin e6-linked drug delivery system co-loaded with cisplatin and metformin for the treatment of head and neck squamous cell carcinoma. The photosensitizer chlorin e6 showed laser-triggered photothermal therapy and photodynamic therapy effects, while cisplatin and metformin served as the chemotherapeutic core [47].

A novel near-infrared-triggered drug release system for combined photothermal therapy, photodynamic therapy, and chemotherapy was investigated by Wang et al. [48]. Nanoparticles were formed using human serum albumin, indocyanine green (Figure 3) and cisplatin. The nanoparticles ensured site-specific drug delivery/release and reduced chemotherapy's systemic toxicity, demonstrating the synergistic effects of photodynamic therapy, photothermal therapy, and chemotherapy with in vitro and in vivo experiments.

Therapeutic protocols for head and neck cancer usually involve chemotherapy, radiotherapy, and/or immunotherapy. Combination therapy is a common trend in oncology. By using various carriers, researchers have proposed a multimodal treatment approach combining chemotherapy and optical therapy, which seem to be beneficial in treating oral cancer [48].

Wang et al. [49] developed novel nanoplatforms for the photothermal therapy of oral cancer with Rose Bengal (Figure 3) as a photodynamic agent and gold nanorods as a photothermal agent. Green laser light was used to activate Rose Bengal, and red laser light for gold nanorods, during an in vitro study with Cal-27 cells. In a study with hamster cheek pouches, an animal model, they found that Rose Bengal–gold nanorods, for combined photodynamic therapy and photothermal therapy, can provide enhanced anti-cancer efficacy against oral cancer. In addition, nanoparticles combined with a laser can be effectively used in photothermal therapy, attacking tumor cells without significant damage to other cells [49].

Ren et al. [50] synthesized hybrid nanoparticles composed of poly(ethylene glycol)-polycaprolactone, with incorporated organic compound (C3) and indocyanine green as photothermal therapy and photodynamic therapy agents, respectively. This nanoplatform was able to simultaneously produce hyperthermia through C3 and produce reactive oxygen species and a fluorescence-guided effect through indocyanine green to kill oral squamous cell carcinoma cells [50].

Another example of a theranostic system developed to treat head and neck squamous cell carcinoma was a combination of photodynamic therapy with gene therapy. The efficacy of photodynamic therapy can be improved by inhibiting the Wnt/β-catenin signaling pathway, which is involved in the activation of the epithelial-to-mesenchymal transition. This transition can lead to tumor recurrence and progression. Ma et al. [51] efficiently delivered siRNA targeting Wnt-1 into the cytoplasm of photodynamic-therapy-treated oral cancer cells using poly(ethylene glycol)-polyethyleneimine-chlorin e6 nanoparticles. This treatment significantly inhibited oral squamous carcinoma cell growth and enhanced the killing effect on cancer cells [51].

8. Targeting Cancer Cells

Although the intravenous administration of photosensitizers has been employed in most clinical trials, the potential side effects should be alleviated. Among the problems of photodynamic therapy are tissue selectivity for the photosensitizers, tissue hypoxia, and tissue penetration of light [52]. The main side effect of photodynamic therapy is systemic, off-target photosensitization resulting from the intravenous administration of the photosensitizer [53,54]. Thus, the intratumoral delivery of the photosensitizer in liposomes, and the potential retention of the liposomes locally via the liposome design, will be highly advantageous. We envision that photosensitizer-encapsulating liposomes can be injected directly, targeting the liposomes to markers overexpressed in cancer cells and will minimize delivery to normal cells around the malignant lesion. Another disadvantage of photodynamic therapy is the necessity to direct the light source to the tumor. Thus, the primary indication for this therapy is in the treatment of superficial and easily accessible cancers [54]. The intravenous injection of the Foscan formulation of mTHPC is painful, results in severe weight loss and acute liver toxicity in CAL-33 tumor-bearing nude mice, whereas the Lipidot nano-emulsion does not cause these side-effects [55], indicating that an association with a lipidic carrier can alleviate some of the toxic effects of photosensitizers. However, this method still does not overcome the systemic photosensitivity of the treated patient.

Although the direct delivery of photosensitizers into oral squamous cell carcinoma lesions may be possible, photocytotoxicity to normal cells surrounding the cancer cells is a side-effect that should ideally be avoided. Using flow cytometry, we examined the binding of fluorescent epidermal growth factor (EGF) to EGF receptors on the surface of HSC-3 human oral squamous cell carcinoma cells, and control, non-tumor-derived GMSM-K cells (Figure 4). We observed extensive binding of EGF to HSC-3 cells and minimal binding to GMSM-K cells, even at 60 min. Confocal fluorescence microscopy showed the extensive internalization of fluorescein-labeled EGF by HSC-3 oral squamous cell carcinoma cells (Figure 5). These observations can be extended to the use of photosensitizer-incorporating liposomes with EGF or anti-EGF receptor antibodies attached covalently to their surface.

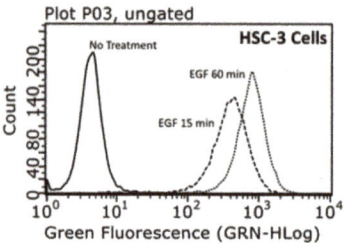

(a)

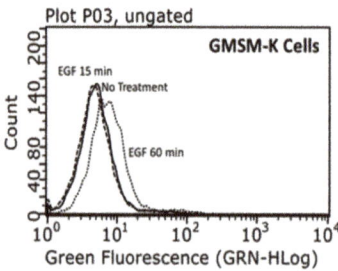

(b)

Figure 4. Flow cytometry of EGF binding to HSC-3 (**a**) and control GMSM-K cells (**b**).

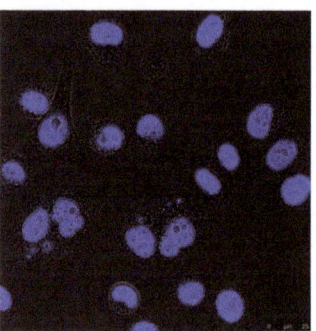 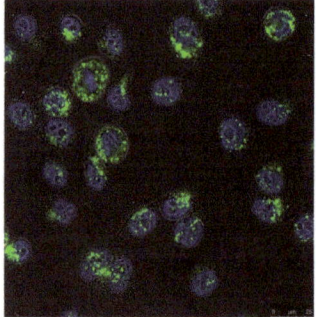

Figure 5. Confocal fluorescence microscopy of fluorescein-labeled EGF internalized by HSC-3 cells following a 15 min incubation with 1 µg/mL EGF. **Left** panel: untreated cells with Hoechst dye; **Right** panel: treated cells.

9. Novel Porphyrinoids with High In Vitro Cytotoxic Activity against Oral Cancer Cells

9.1. Sulfanyl Porphyrazines with Fluoroalkyl and Diether Chains

Our laboratories have been working on the development of novel photosensitizers and their photocytotoxicity on oral cancer cells. Two sulfanyl porphyrazines, possessing 4-fluorobutyl (**1a**) and 2-(2-ethoxyethoxy)ethyl (**1b**) substituents (Figure 6), were studied using human oral squamous cell carcinoma cell lines derived from the tongue (HSC-3) and the buccal mucosa (H413) [56]. Porphyrazines **1a,b** in the concentration range 1–50 μM showed no dark toxicity, i.e., without light exposure. At 50 μM, however, both **1a** and **1b** aggregated, as noted under the microscope.

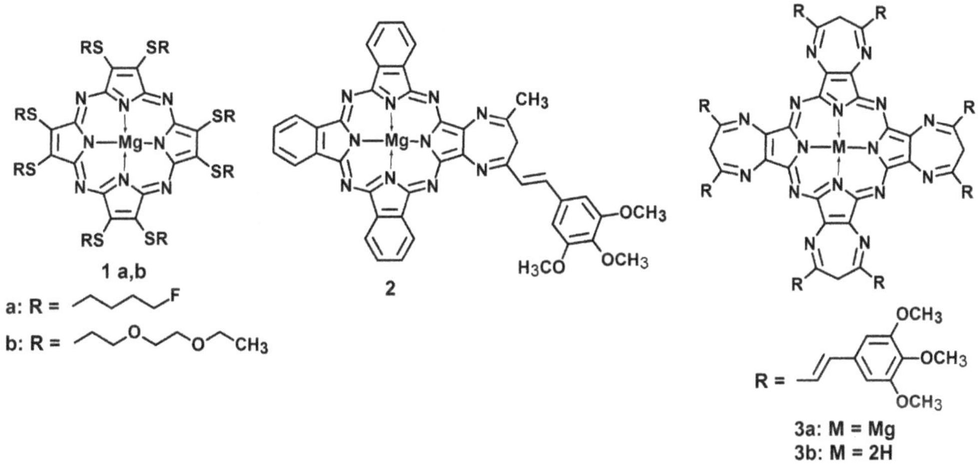

Figure 6. The chemical structure of porphyrazines **1**–**3**.

The light-induced toxicity was tested at 1 and 5 μM after exposure to light of 600–850 nm. No light-induced toxicity was observed for porphyrazine **1b** on both cell lines, and for **1a** for HSC-3 cells. By contrast, **1a** reduced the H413 cell viability by about 30–35% at both concentrations. Thus, the phototoxicity of the sulfanyl porphyrazine with fluoroalkyl substituents was found to be cell-dependent, although these cells are derived from the same type of tumor.

9.2. Porphyrazines and Tribenzoporphyrazine with Annulated Diazepine Rings

Further studies using HSC-3 and H413 cells were performed with porphyrazines and tribenzoporphyrazine possessing annulated diazepine rings (**2**, **3**, Figure 6) [57]. Dark toxicity experiments in the concentration range 0.1–10 μM showed that only tribenzoporphyrazine **2** on H413 cells showed some dark toxicity at concentrations higher than 1 μM. Photocytotoxicity studies after LED light irradiation at 690 nm revealed that the viability of the H413 cells was reduced by 90% at 1.0 μM of compound **2**, and by **3a** at 10 μM by about 25%, whereas **3b** did not show any significant viability reduction. In the case of HSC-3 cells, a photocytotoxic effect of about 95% was found for compound **2** at 1 μM and 87% for 10 μM of **3b**. There was no significant reduction in HSC-3 cell viability by porphyrazine **3b**.

The photodynamic efficiency of compounds **2** and **3b** toward HSC-3 cells was also examined after incorporation into four different liposome formulations: (i) L-α-phosphatidyl-D,L-glycerol (PG, from chicken eggs):1-palmitoyl-2-oleoyl-sn-glycero-3-phosphocholine (POPC), (ii) PG:POPC:cholesterol (Chol), (iii) N-[1-(2,3-dioleoyloxy)-propyl]-N,N,N-trimeth-ylammonium chloride (DOTAP):POPC, and (iv) DOTAP:POPC:Chol. All four liposomes containing tribenzoporphyrazine **2** showed high light-induced photodynamic activity [57]. On the contrary, there was no significant photocytotoxic effect of liposomal compound **3b**. The IC_{50} calculations of the four types of liposomes with **2** revealed that the negatively charged liposomes composed of **2**:PG:POPC were the most active. Moreover, their activity was about three times higher than the free form of photosensitizer **2**, indicating that these liposomes are the most potent delivery systems for this photosensitizer.

9.3. Potential Methods of Liposome Administration

We envisage liposomal photosensitizers to be administered in several ways. Analogous to our studies on the injection of suicide genes complexed to transferrin-associated cationic liposomes into orthotopic oral squamous cell carcinoma tumors in mice that result in the arrest of tumor growth following the delivery of the prodrug, ganciclovir [58], they can be injected directly into the tumors. This method may be enhanced by the simultaneous delivery of agents that degrade the tumor microenvironment, enabling the liposomes easier access to the entire tumor. Liu et al. [59] employed collagenase, encapsulated in pH-responsive nanoscale coordination polymers that released their enzyme in the mildly acidic medium of the tumor microenvironment, resulting in a loosened extracellular matrix structure, enhanced tumor perfusion, and relieved hypoxia. They showed that liposomal chlorin-e6 mediated more effective photodynamic therapy following collagenase treatment. Kohli et al. [60] reported that the distribution of liposomal doxorubicin in the tumor matrix was improved after the depletion of tumor hyaluronan. Concerns about the induction of metastases following enzyme treatment have not been borne out [61]. Liposomal photosensitizers may be administered transmucosally by enabling their stable adhesion to the mucosa [62], for example, by the use of cationic liposomes (vide infra). Liposomes may also be potentially embedded in oral films to facilitate their transmucosal transport [63].

9.4. Sulfanyl Porphyrazines with 4-Bromobenzyl and 4-Biphenylylmethyl Substituents

The photocytotoxic effects of free and liposome-encapsulated sulfanyl porphyrazines containing 4-bromobenzyl (**4a**) and 4-biphenylylmethyl substituents (**4b**, Figure 7), on oral cancer cells derived from the tongue (CAL 27, HSC-3), and HeLa human cervical epithelial adenocarcinoma cells, was investigated [64].The photosensitizers in free form did not have any significant photocytotoxicity on any of the cells. The liposomal formulations of these porphyrazines were prepared using two different types of nanoparticles, composed of PG:POPC or DOTAP:POPC. Porphyrazine **4a**, incorporated into the positively charged DOTAP:POPC liposomes, showed high photocytotoxicity with the reduction in the cell viability by about 90% at 10 µM. The viability of cells at 1 µm was decreased by 47% for HSC-3 and 34% for CAL 27 cells. There was no significant reduction in the HeLa cell viability. The phototoxicity of liposomal formulations containing the biphenylyl analog **4b** was much lower. Cationic DOTAP:POPC liposomes showed light-induced toxicity against HSC-3 cells, reducing cell viability by about 30% at 10 µM, but not against other cells. The negatively charged **4b**:PG:POPC liposomes did not have any photocytotoxicity. The results indicated that DOTAP:POPC liposomes could be a promising drug delivery system for sulfanyl porphyrazines, but their effectiveness also depends on the photosensitizer structure.

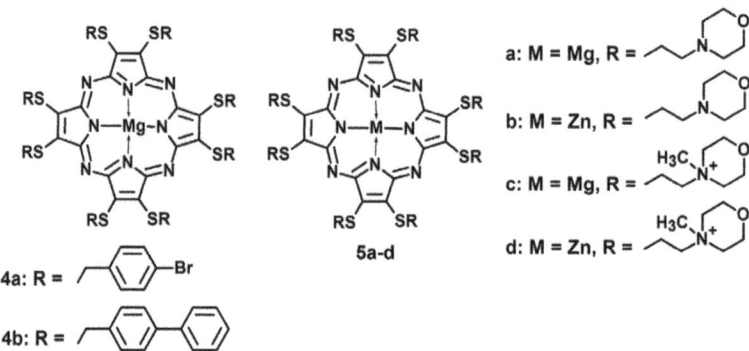

Figure 7. The chemical structure of porphyrazines **4,5**.

9.5. Sulfanyl Porphyrazines with Morpholinoethyl and N-Methylmorpholinoethyl Substituents

Magnesium(II) and zinc(II) porphyrazines, bearing morpholinoethyl (**5a,b**) and cationic N-methylmorpholinoethyl substituents (**5c,d**, Figure 7), were tested on squamous cell carcinoma cell lines SCC-25 and CAL-27 derived from the tongue [65]. They were tested in free forms administered to the cell culture medium in the range 0.01–5.0 µM, and in POPC:POPG (1-palmitoyl-2-oleoyl-sn-glycero-3-phospho-1′-rac-glycerol sodium salt) liposomes at 0.01–2.0 µM. Despite their similar origin, CAL 27 cells were found to be less susceptible to photodynamic treatment than SCC-25 cells. Magnesium(II) porphyrazine, with morpholinoethyl groups (**5a**), showed high photocytotoxicity on both cell lines, with IC_{50} values of 0.75 and 1.20 µM for SCC-25 and CAL 27 cells, respectively. In addition, the liposomal formulation of **5a** was even more active, with IC_{50} = 0.64 µM for SCC-25 and 0.69 µM for CAL 27 cells. The zinc analog **5b** revealed lower effectiveness, with the phototoxic effect observed only against SCC-cells (IC_{50} = 6.46 µM), which increased almost twice after liposomal incorporation (IC_{50} = 3.61 µM). However, porphyrazines containing cationic N-methylmorpholinoethyl substituents (**5c,d**) did not show any significant cytotoxicity on tested cancer cells.

9.6. Sulfanyl Tribenzoporphyrazines with Dendrimeric Moieties

Sulfanyl tribenzoporphyrazines were another important subgroup of photosensitizers subjected to studies against oral cancer cells. Three such macrocycles with dendrimeric moieties (**6a–c**, Figure 8) were tested on CAL 27 and HSC-3 cells [66]. After being exposed to LED light of 690 nm, all three photosensitizers showed a photocytotoxic effect against tested cells. Tribenzoporphyrazine **6a** with branched G_1-dendrimeric substituents showed moderate activity toward CAL 27 cells with an IC_{50} value of 3.13 µM, but much higher activity against HSC-3 cells (IC_{50} = 0.64 µM). The decrease in the dendrimeric substituent generation to G_0 in the case of tribenzoporphyrazine **6b** resulted in reduced photocytotoxicity, as the IC_{50} values reached 6.66 and 10.6 µM for CAL 27 and HSC-3 cells, respectively. However, the lowest nanomolar IC_{50} values of 10 nM for CAL 27 and 42 nM for HSC-3 were reached by **6c**, in whose structure butoxycarbonyl substituents were reduced to hydroxymethyl groups. In further studies, porphyrazine **6b** was subjected to an oxidation reaction, resulting in the oxidative breaking of the one pyrrole ring and the formation of the S-seco-tribenzoporphyrazine analogue **7** (Figure 8) [66]. The photodynamic activity of the seco-derivative **7** on CAL 27 and HSC-3 cells was very potent, with IC_{50} values of 0.61 and 0.18 µM, respectively. This activity was much higher than those for the precursor **6b**.

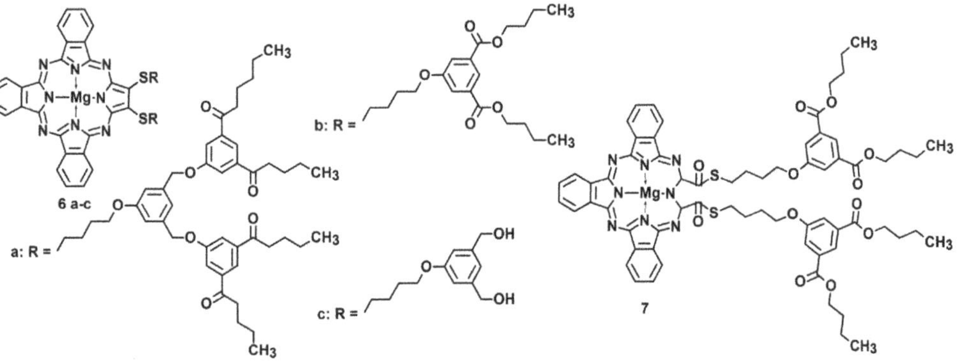

Figure 8. The chemical structure of porphyrazines **6,7**.

Photosensitizers **6a–c** and **7** were also tested after incorporating them into four liposomal formulations [67,68]. Zwitterionic lipids POPC or 1,2-dioleoyl-sn-glycero-3-phosphoethanolamine (DOPE) constituted the main components of the liposomes, whereas PG or DOTAP were added to provide a negative or positive charge, respectively. For all tested tribenzoporphyrazines, cationic DOTAP:POPC liposomes had the highest photodynamic activity. Notably, the IC_{50} values for this formulation were up to 50 times lower compared to the free forms of tribenzoporphyrazines, and the oral cancer cells, CAL 27 and HSC-3, were more sensitive to photodynamic treatment than the HeLa cervical adenocarcinoma cells.

9.7. Phthalocyanines

Phthalocyanines constitute another class of porphyrinoids that we tested on oral cancer cells. Two commercially available compounds, zinc phthalocyanine (ZnPc) and aluminum phthalocyanine chloride (AlPc, Figure 9), were examined on HSC-3 and HeLa cells [69]. The photosensitizers were prepared in free forms dissolved in the culture medium, as well as incorporated into negatively charged PG:POPC liposomes. Both phthalocyanines revealed a phototoxic effect, which was dependent on cell type. Zinc phthalocyanine was more effective against HSC-3 cells, whose viability was reduced to 22% at 1.0 μM photosensitizer, whereas the viability of HeLa cells decreased to 53% at the same concentration of ZnPc. By contrast, HeLa cells were more sensitive to the treatment with aluminum phthalocyanine chloride. The viability of cells after photodynamic treatment with 1.0 μM of AlPc decreased to 15 and 57% for HeLa and HSC-3 cells, respectively. Moreover, liposomal incorporation enhanced the cytotoxic effect of both phthalocyanines. A lethal photodynamic effect on both cell types was observed for liposomes containing 1.0 μM of ZnPc, while AlPc-liposomes at the same concentration caused a lethal effect on HeLa cells, but the viability of HSC-3 cells was reduced to only 21%.

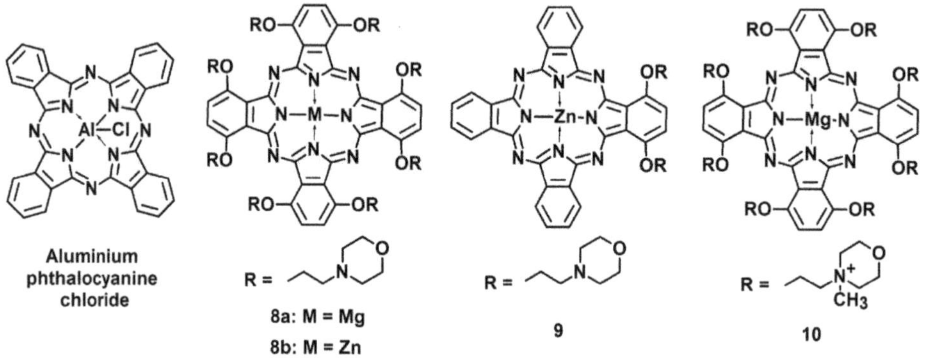

Figure 9. The chemical structure of AlPc and phthalocyanines **8–10**.

In another study, zinc phthalocyanine was incorporated in two types of liposomes composed of POPG:POPC or POPG:DOPE [70]. The photodynamic activity of obtained liposomes, both extruded and non-extruded, was tested on CAL27 cells and FaDu pharyngeal carcinoma cells. Surprisingly, POPG:DOPE liposomes did not have photocytotoxicity against tested cell lines. On the other hand, zinc phthalocyanine in free form, and incorporated into extruded POPG:POPC liposomes, showed a significant photodynamic effect, which was higher on CAL 27 cells, compared to FaDu cells. The ZnPc, dissolved in culture medium at 0.1 and 0.5 μM concentrations, decreased the viability of CAL 27 cells by about 20% and 70%, respectively. The viability of FaDu cells was not affected at 0.1 μM and reduced by about 60% at 0.5 μM. The incorporation of ZnPc in extruded POPG:POPC liposomes resulted in highly increased photocytotoxicity; at 0.1 and 0.5 μM concentrations, a lethal effect was observed on CAL 27 cells. In the case of HeLa cells, a 0.5 μM concentration was also lethal, but, at 0.1 μM, cell viability was decreased to 6%.

Novel phthalocyanines synthesized by our team were also examined on oral cancer cells. Magnesium and zinc phthalocyanines (**8a, b**), as well as zinc tribenzoporphyrazine (**9**) containing 2-(morpholin-4-yl)ethoxy substituents (Figure 9), were examined on HSC-3 and

H413 cancer cells derived from the tongue and buccal mucosa, respectively [71]. Tribenzoporphyrazine **9** definitely showed the highest photocytotoxic effect. However, significant dark toxicity was observed with H413 cells, reaching 21 and 74% at 1.0 and 10 µM concentrations. HSC-3 cells were unaffected by **9** in this concentration range in the dark, while, after irradiation, the cell viability was reduced by >90% and >80% at 0.1 and 1.0 µM. Photosensitizers **8a**, **b**, and **9** were also incorporated into PG:POPC and DOTAP:POPC liposomes, but, surprisingly, they did not strongly affect biological activity against HSC-3 and H413 cells. Another study on HSC3 and H413 cells involved phthalocyanine containing cationic N-methylmorpholiniumethoxy substituents (**10**, Figure 9) in free form and incorporated into PG:POPC liposomes [72]. Surprisingly, besides a high photodynamic activity against both Gram-positive and Gram-negative bacteria, no significant photocytotoxicity toward oral cancer cells was observed.

9.8. Other Porphyrinoid Photosensitizers

The photodynamic activity of other porphyrinoid photosensitizers on various cancer cells has been examined recently, both in free forms and in drug delivery systems, including liposomal formulations [5,73,74]. However, the reports concerning oral cancer cells are very limited. Thomas et al. [75] investigated the photosensitizing activity of a water-soluble N-confused porphyrin with 4-sulfonatophenyl substituents on oral squamous cell carcinoma cell lines SCC-131 (IC$_{50}$ = 13 µM) and SCC-172 (IC$_{50}$ = 11 µM) [75]. Chin and coworkers studied the photodynamic activity of three glycerol substituted phthalocyanines on MCF-7 breast carcinoma, HCT-116 colon carcinoma, and HSC-2 oral squamous cell carcinoma cells. Non-peripherally tetra-glycerol-substituted and mono-iodo tri-glycerol-substituted phthalocyanines showed promising activity with IC$_{50}$ values in the range of 2.8–3.2 µM and 0.04–0.06 µM for tetra-glycerol and mono-iodo tri-glycerol analogs, respectively [76]. A chlorin-based photosensitizer, pheophorbide a, was used on YD10B and YD38 oral squamous cell carcinoma cell lines [77]. The viability of YD10B cells decreased by 70% after treatment, and that of YD38 cells by 60%. A greater increase in ROS generation, and in the number of apoptotic cells, were also observed for YD10B cells compared to the YD38 cells. Moreover, the RUNX3 gene related to apoptosis was selected as a potential marker for determining sensitivity to photodynamic therapy with pheophorbide a. It was found that the expression level of RUNX3 was proportional to the percentage of PDT-induced cell death [77]. Chu and coworkers [78] studied the effect of vandetanib, a blocker of epidermal growth factor receptor (EGFR) and vascular endothelial growth factor receptor-2 (VEGFR-2), on the efficiency of photodynamic therapy. The studies performed with Chlorin e6 on CAL 27 oral cancer cells revealed that adding vandetanib enhanced photocytotoxicity. This result was explained by both the direct and indirect effects of vandetanib on the cellular DNA repair machinery and tumor microenvironment [78].

10. Future Directions in the Photodynamic Therapy of Oral Cancer

10.1. Targeting Photosensitizers to Cancer Stem Cells

Cancer stem cells are a small subpopulation of existing tumors or cancer cells that can regenerate the original tumor or cancer, first recognized in leukemia [79,80]. Cancer stem cells have also been identified in head and neck squamous cell carcinoma [81–83]. Although CD44 is a surface marker for cancer stem cells, it is not entirely specific. Cells that express both CD44 and CD271 upregulate cancer stem-cell related genes and show higher tumorigenicity than cells expressing only CD44 [84]. These observations raise the possibility of targeting photosensitizers embedded in or encapsulated inside liposomes via the use of antibodies against CD44 and against CD271, similar to the example given above with epidermal growth factor.

10.2. Upconversion Nanoparticles for Near-Infrared Irradiation of Tumors

The absorption wavelengths of the photosensitizers used in photodynamic therapy are too short to enable sufficient tissue penetration to reach cells located deeper in tumors.

Upconversion involves the generation of high-energy (shorter wavelength) light from near-infrared, low-energy radiation that can reach deeper tissues [85,86]. As a case in point, Sawamura et al. [87] used nanoparticles composed of a lanthanide, which, upon excitation with near-infrared light (980 nm), emits light of wavelengths in the Soret band (405 nm), and one of the a Q bands (540 nm), of the photosensitizer, protoporphyrin IX PPIX. The lanthanide nanoparticles were derivatized with amino groups to bind to the human gastric cancer cell line, MKN45, and irradiation of the system with near-infrared light caused extensive cytotoxicity. Chlorin e6 complexed with upconversion lanthanide nanoparticles that emit in the ultraviolet, blue, and red regions when excited at 980 nm had a significant cytotoxic effect on MCF-7 human breast cancer cells cultured as tumor spheroids [88]. This effect was stronger than that induced by irradiation at 660 nm.

10.3. Overcoming Tumor Hypoxia

The tumor microenvironment exhibits acidic pH and hypoxia resulting from the high metabolic activity of dividing cancer cells. The oxygen tension (pO$_2$) in tumors is usually less than 5 mmHg, whereas it is in the range 10 to 80 mmHg in normal tissue [89]. The therapeutic effect of type-II photodynamic therapy is such that the photosensitizers in the triplet state transfer their energy directly to $^3O_2$ to produce singlet oxygen ($^1O_2$). This process obviously requires the presence of O$_2$, and thus, increasing the O$_2$ concentration of the tumor is likely to enhance the efficacy of photodynamic therapy. Some of the methods to counter tumor hypoxia are to introduce exogenous O$_2$ to the tumor, generate de novo O$_2$ in the tumor, degrade the tumor microenvironment, and inhibit the signaling pathway for hypoxia-inducible factor 1 (HIF-1) [89].

11. Conclusions

Current standard treatments for squamous cell carcinoma of the head and neck are inadequate. Photodynamic therapy may be advantageous over conventional treatments because of its minimal invasiveness, its selective tumor destruction and, thus, the preservation of healthy tissues. Some photosensitizers may localize preferentially in tumors, and liposomes carrying photosensitizers may be targeted to receptors overexpressed on certain cancer cells to mediate a much higher accumulation of the photosensitizer compared to normal cells. The use of Foscan in the treatment of early oral squamous cell carcinoma resulted in a response rate of 93% for T1 lesions and 58% for T2 lesions. In a group of 170 patients with early-stage oral cavity and oropharynx squamous cell cancers or carcinoma in situ, treated with intravenous Foscan followed by light exposure, an overall response rate of 91%, and a complete response rate of 71%, were obtained. The theranostic approach to the delivery of photosensitizers integrates imaging and stimuli-responsive therapeutic delivery within one system. One example of this approach is poly(ethylene glycol)-polycaprolactone nanoparticles containing the organic compound, C3, for photothermal therapy, and indocyanine green for photodynamic therapy to kill oral squamous cell carcinoma cells. We have synthesized and tested the anti-cancer activities of derivatives of sulfany porphyrazines, sulfanyl tribenzoporphyrazine, porphyrazines, and tribenzoporphyrazines, both as free drugs and incorporated in the liposome membrane. Tribenzoporphyrazines encapsulated in positively charged liposomes exhibited the highest photodynamic activity, with IC$_{50}$ values up to 50 times lower compared to the free forms of the drugs. Thus, the avid binding of these photosensitizers to oral cancer cells, and their internalization, enables a much higher photocytotoxicity. Current and future studies on targeting liposomal photosensitizers to oral cancer cells, on the generation of liposomes or other nanoparticles enabling deeper penetration of near-infrared irradiation of tumors, and on the generation of local oxygen in tumors, are highly likely to enhance our ability to treat oral premalignant or cancerous lesions.

Author Contributions: J.P., P.S.-M., M.Y., M.S. and N.D. wrote the manuscript and edited it. J.P. contributed figures and J.C. contributed data. All authors have read and agreed to the published version of the manuscript.

Funding: No external funding was used in the writing of this article.

Institutional Review Board Statement: Not applicable.

Informed Consent Statement: Not applicable.

Data Availability Statement: All data are available in the manuscript.

Conflicts of Interest: The authors declare no conflict of interest.

References

1. Mouth and Oral Cancer Statistics. Available online: https://www.wcrf.org/cancer-trends/mouth-and-oral-cancer-statistics (accessed on 26 January 2023).
2. Abrahamse, H.; Hamblin, M.R. New photosensitizers for photodynamic therapy. *Biochem. J.* **2016**, *473*, 347–364. [CrossRef] [PubMed]
3. Melissari, Z.; Sample, H.C.; Twamley, B.; Williams, R.M.; Senge, M.O. Synthesis and spectral properties of gem-dimethyl chlorin photosensitizers. *Chemphotochem* **2020**, *4*, 601–611. [CrossRef]
4. Yao, Q.C.; Fan, J.L.; Long, S.R.; Zhao, X.Z.; Li, H.D.; Du, J.J.; Shao, K.; Peng, X.J. The concept and examples of type-III photosensitizers for cancer photodynamic therapy. *Chem* **2022**, *8*, 197–209. [CrossRef]
5. Rak, J.; Kabesova, M.; Benes, J.; Pouckova, P.; Vetvicka, D. Advances in liposome-encapsulated phthalocyanines for photodynamic therapy. *Life* **2023**, *13*, 305. [CrossRef]
6. Skupin-Mrugalska, P.; Sobotta, L.; Kucinska, M.; Murias, M.; Mielcarek, J.; Düzgüneş, N. Cellular changes, molecular pathways and the immune system following photodynamic treatment. *Curr. Med. Chem.* **2014**, *21*, 4059–4073. [CrossRef]
7. Chen, H.M.; Liu, C.M.; Yang, H.; Chou, H.Y.; Chiang, C.P.; Kuo, M.Y. 5-aminolevulinic acid induce apoptosis via NF-kappaB/JNK pathway in human oral cancer Ca9-22 cells. *J. Oral Pathol. Med.* **2011**, *40*, 483–489. [CrossRef] [PubMed]
8. Ahn, M.Y.; Yoon, H.E.; Kwon, S.M.; Lee, J.; Min, S.K.; Kim, Y.C.; Ahn, S.G.; Yoon, J.H. Synthesized Pheophorbide a-mediated photodynamic therapy induced apoptosis and autophagy in human oral squamous carcinoma cells. *J. Oral Pathol. Med.* **2013**, *42*, 17–25. [CrossRef] [PubMed]
9. Alzeibak, R.; Mishchenko, T.A.; Shilyagina, N.Y. Targeting immunogenic cancer cell death by photodynamic therapy: Past, present and future. *J. Immunother. Cancer* **2021**, *9*, e001926. [CrossRef] [PubMed]
10. Konopka, K.; Goslinski, T. Photodynamic therapy in dentistry. *J. Dent. Res.* **2007**, *86*, 694–707. [CrossRef]
11. Wooten, R.S.; Ahlquist, D.A.; Anderson, R.E.; Carpenter, H.A.; Pemberton, J.H.; Cortese, D.A.; Ilstrup, D.M. Localization of hematoporphyrin. Derivative to human colorectal cancer. *Cancer* **1989**, *64*, 1569–1576. [CrossRef]
12. Dougherty, T.J.; Gomer, C.J.; Henderson, B.W.; Jori, G.; Kessel, D.; Korbelik, M.; Moan, J.; Peng, Q. Photodynamic therapy. *J. Natl. Cancer Inst.* **1998**, *90*, 889–905. [CrossRef]
13. Wang, Z.J.; He, Y.Y.; Huang, C.G.; Huang, J.S.; Huang, Y.C.; An, J.Y.; Gu, Y.; Jiang, L.J. Pharmacokinetics, tissue distribution and photodynamic therapy efficacy of liposomal-delivered hypocrellin A, a potential photosensitizer for tumor therapy. *Photochem. Photobiol.* **1999**, *70*, 773–780. [CrossRef]
14. Derycke, A.S.; de Witte, P.A. Liposomes for photodynamic therapy. *Adv. Drug Deliv. Rev.* **2004**, *56*, 17–30. [CrossRef]
15. Biel, M.A. Photodynamic therapy in head and neck cancer. *Curr. Oncol. Rep.* **2002**, *4*, 87–96. [CrossRef]
16. Fukuda, H.; Casas, A.; Batlle, A. Aminolevulinic acid: From its unique biological function to its star role in photodynamic therapy. *Int. J. Biochem. Cell Biol.* **2005**, *37*, 272–276. [CrossRef]
17. Chen, Q.; Dan, H.; Tang, F.; Wang, J.; Li, X.; Cheng, J.; Zhao, H.; Zeng, X. Photodynamic therapy guidelines for the management of oral leucoplakia. *Int. J. Oral Sci.* **2019**, *11*, 14. [CrossRef]
18. Wong, S.J.; Campbell, B.; Massey, B.; Lynch, D.P.; Cohen, E.E.W.; Blair, E.; Selle, R.; Shklovskaya, J.; Jovanovic, B.D.; Skripkauskas, S.; et al. A phase I trial of aminolevulinic acid-photodynamic therapy for treatment of oral leukoplakia. *Oral Oncol.* **2013**, *49*, 970–976. [CrossRef] [PubMed]
19. Kubler, A.; Haase, T.; Rheinwald, M.; Barth, T.; Muhling, J. Treatment of oral leukoplakia by topical application of 5-aminolevulinic acid. *Int. J. Oral Maxillofac. Surg.* **1998**, *27*, 466–469. [CrossRef]
20. Sieron, A.; Adamek, M.; Kawczyk-Krupka, A.; Mazur, S.; Ilewicz, L. Photodynamic therapy (PDT) using topically applied delta-aminolevulinic acid (ALA) for the treatment of oral leukoplakia. *J. Oral Pathol. Med.* **2003**, *32*, 330–336. [CrossRef]
21. Chen, H.M.; Yu, C.H.; Tu, P.C.; Yeh, C.Y.; Tsai, T.; Chiang, C.P. Successful treatment of oral verrucous hyperplasia and oral leukoplakia with topical 5-aminolevulinic acid-mediated photodynamic therapy. *Lasers Surg. Med.* **2005**, *37*, 114–122. [CrossRef]
22. Siddiqui, S.A.; Siddiqui, S.; Hussain, M.A.B.; Khan, S.; Liu, H.; Akhtar, K.; Hasan, S.A.; Ahmed, I.; Mallidi, S.; Khan, A.P.; et al. Clinical evaluation of a mobile, low-cost system for fluorescence guided photodynamic therapy of early oral cancer in India. *Photodiagnosis Photodyn. Ther.* **2022**, *38*, 102843. [CrossRef]
23. Yao, Y.L.; Wang, Y.F.; Li, C.X.; Wu, L.; Tang, G.Y. Management of oral leukoplakia by ablative fractional laser-assisted photodynamic therapy: A 3-year retrospective study of 48 patients. *Lasers Surg. Med.* **2022**, *54*, 682–687. [CrossRef]
24. Gorsky, M.; Epstein, J.B. Oral lichen planus: Malignant transformation and human papilloma virus: A review of potential clinical implications. *Oral Surg. Oral Med. Oral Pathol. Oral Radiol. Endod.* **2011**, *111*, 461–464. [CrossRef]

25. Raghavendra Kini, D.N.; Saha, A. Therapeutic Management of Oral Lichen Planus: A Review for the Clinicians. *World J. Dent.* **2011**, *2*, 249–253. [CrossRef]
26. Tardivo, J.P.; Del Giglio, A.; de Oliveira, C.S.; Gabrielli, D.S.; Junqueira, H.C.; Tada, D.B.; Severino, D.; de Fatima Turchiello, R.; Baptista, M.S. Methylene blue in photodynamic therapy: From basic mechanisms to clinical applications. *Photodiagnosis Photodyn. Ther.* **2005**, *2*, 175–191. [CrossRef]
27. Aghahosseini, F.; Arbabi-Kalati, F.; Fashtami, L.A.; Djavid, G.E.; Fateh, M.; Beitollahi, J.M. Methylene blue-mediated photodynamic therapy: A possible alternative treatment for oral lichen planus. *Lasers Surg. Med.* **2006**, *38*, 33–38. [CrossRef]
28. Sadaksharam, J.; Nayaki, K.P.; Selvam, N.P. Treatment of oral lichen planus with methylene blue mediated photodynamic therapy—A clinical study. *Photodermatol. Photoimmunol. Photomed.* **2012**, *28*, 97–101. [CrossRef]
29. Bakhtiari, S.; Azari-Marhabi, S.; Mojahedi, S.M.; Namdari, M.; Rankohi, Z.E.; Jafari, S. Comparing clinical effects of photodynamic therapy as a novel method with topical corticosteroid for treatment of oral lichen planus. *Photodiagnosis Photodyn. Ther.* **2017**, *20*, 159–164. [CrossRef]
30. Mostafa, D.; Moussa, E.; Alnouaem, M. Evaluation of photodynamic therapy in treatment of oral erosive lichen planus in comparison with topically applied corticosteroids. *Photodiagnosis Photodyn. Ther.* **2017**, *19*, 56–66. [CrossRef]
31. Biel, M.A. Photodynamic therapy and the treatment of head and neck cancers. *J. Clin. Laser Med. Surg.* **1996**, *14*, 239–244. [CrossRef]
32. Biel, M.A. Photodynamic therapy as an adjuvant intraoperative treatment of recurrent head and neck carcinomas. *Arch. Otolaryngol.* **1996**, *122*, 1261–1265. [CrossRef] [PubMed]
33. Biel, M. Advances in photodynamic therapy for the treatment of head and neck cancers. *Lasers Surg. Med.* **2006**, *38*, 349–355. [CrossRef] [PubMed]
34. Ikeda, H.; Tobita, T.; Ohba, S.; Uehara, M.; Asahina, I. Treatment outcome of Photofrin-based photodynamic therapy for T1 and T2 oral squamous cell carcinoma and dysplasia. *Photodiagnosis Photodyn. Ther.* **2013**, *10*, 229–235. [CrossRef] [PubMed]
35. Hopper, C.; Kubler, A.; Lewis, H.; Tan, I.B.; Putnam, G. mTHPC-mediated photodynamic therapy for early oral squamous cell carcinoma. *Int. J. Cancer* **2004**, *111*, 138–146. [CrossRef]
36. D'Cruz, A.K.; Robinson, M.H.; Biel, M.A. mTHPC-mediated photodynamic therapy in patients with advanced, incurable head and neck cancer: A multicenter study of 128 patients. *Head Neck* **2004**, *26*, 232–240. [CrossRef] [PubMed]
37. Kubler, A.C.; de Carpentier, J.; Hopper, C.; Leonard, A.G.; Putnam, G. Treatment of squamous cell carcinoma of the lip using Foscan-mediated photodynamic therapy. *Int. J. Oral Maxillofac. Surg* **2001**, *30*, 504–509. [CrossRef]
38. Kubler, A.; Niziol, C.; Sidhu, M.; Dunne, A.; Werner, J.A. Analysis of cost effectiveness of photodynamic therapy with Foscan (Foscan-PDT) in comparison with palliative chemotherapy in patients with advanced head-neck tumors in Germany. *Laryngorhinootologie* **2005**, *84*, 725–732. [CrossRef]
39. Karakullukçu, B.; van Oudenaarde, K.; Copper, M.P.; Klop, W.M.; van Veen, R.; Wildeman, M.; Bing Tan, I. Photodynamic therapy of early stage oral cavity and oropharynx neoplasms: An outcome analysis of 170 patients. *Eur. Arch. Otorhinolaryngol.* **2011**, *268*, 281–288. [CrossRef]
40. Copper, M.P.; Tan, I.B.; Oppelaar, H.; Ruevekamp, M.C.; Stewart, F.A. Meta-tetra(hydroxyphenyl)chlorin photodynamic therapy in early-stage squamous cell carcinoma of the head and neck. *Arch. Otolaryngol. Head Neck Surg.* **2003**, *129*, 709–711. [CrossRef]
41. Jerjes, W.; Upile, T.; Radhi, H.; Hopper, C. Photodynamic therapy and end-stage tongue base cancer: Short communication. *Head Neck Oncol.* **2011**, *3*, 49. [CrossRef]
42. Sobaniec, S.; Bernaczyk, P.; Pietruski, J.; Cholewa, M.; Skurska, A.; Dolinska, E.; Duraj, E.; Tokajuk, G.; Paniczko, A.; Olszewska, E.; et al. Clinical assessment of the efficacy of photodynamic therapy in the treatment of oral lichen planus. *Lasers Med. Sci.* **2013**, *28*, 311–316. [CrossRef]
43. Rigual, N.; Shafirstein, G.; Cooper, M.T.; Baumann, H.; Bellnier, D.A.; Sunar, U.; Tracy, E.C.; Rohrbach, D.J.; Wilding, G.; Tan, W.; et al. Photodynamic therapy with 3-(1′-hexyloxyethyl) pyropheophorbide a for cancer of the oral cavity. *Clin. Cancer Res.* **2013**, *19*, 6605–6613. [CrossRef]
44. Skupin-Mrugalska, P.; Zalewski, T.; Elvang, P.A.; Nowaczyk, G.; Czajkowski, M.; Piotrowska-Kempisty, H. Insight into theranostic nanovesicles prepared by thin lipid hydration and microfluidic method. *Colloids Surf. B Biointerfaces* **2021**, *205*, 111871. [CrossRef]
45. Wang, D.; Fei, B.; Halig, L.V.; Qin, X.; Hu, Z.; Xu, H.; Wang, Y.A.; Chen, Z.; Kim, S.; Shin, D.M.; et al. Targeted iron-oxide nanoparticle for photodynamic therapy and imaging of head and neck cancer. *ACS Nano* **2014**, *8*, 6620–6632. [CrossRef]
46. Liang, J.; Yang, B.; Zhou, X.; Han, Q.; Zou, J.; Cheng, L. Stimuli-responsive drug delivery systems for head and neck cancer therapy. *Drug Deliv.* **2021**, *28*, 272–284. [CrossRef]
47. Song, C.; Ran, J.; Wei, Z.; Wang, Y.; Chen, S.; Lin, L.; Zhang, G.; Cai, Y.; Han, W. Organic near-infrared-II nanophotosensitizer for safe cancer phototheranostics and improving immune microenvironment against metastatic tumor. *ACS Appl. Mater. Interfaces* **2021**, *13*, 3547–3558. [CrossRef] [PubMed]
48. Wang, Y.; Xie, D.; Pan, J.; Xia, C.; Fan, L.; Pu, Y.; Zhang, Q.; Ni, Y.H.; Wang, J.; Hu, Q. A near infrared light-triggered human serum albumin drug delivery system with coordination bonding of indocyanine green and cisplatin for targeting photochemistry therapy against oral squamous cell cancer. *Biomater. Sci.* **2019**, *7*, 5270–5282. [CrossRef] [PubMed]
49. Wang, B.; Wang, J.H.; Liu, Q.; Huang, H.; Chen, M.; Li, K.; Li, C.; Yu, X.F.; Chu, P.K. Rose-bengal-conjugated gold nanorods for in vivo photodynamic and photothermal oral cancer therapies. *Biomaterials* **2014**, *35*, 1954–1966. [CrossRef]

50. Ren, S.; Cheng, X.; Chen, M.; Liu, C.; Zhao, P.; Huang, W.; He, J.; Zhou, Z.; Miao, L. Hypotoxic and rapidly metabolic PEG-PCL-C3-ICG nanoparticles for fluorescence-guided photothermal/photodynamic therapy against OSCC. *ACS Appl. Mater. Interfaces* **2017**, *9*, 31509–31518. [CrossRef] [PubMed]
51. Ma, C.; Shi, L.; Huang, Y.; Shen, L.; Peng, H.; Zhu, X.; Zhou, G. Nanoparticle delivery of Wnt-1 siRNA enhances photodynamic therapy by inhibiting epithelial-mesenchymal transition for oral cancer. *Biomater. Sci.* **2017**, *5*, 494–501. [CrossRef] [PubMed]
52. Günaydin, G.; Gedik, M.E.; Ayan, S. Photodynamic therapy-current limitations and novel approaches. *Front. Chem.* **2021**, *9*, 691697. [CrossRef] [PubMed]
53. Jerjes, W.; Hamdoon, Z.; Hopper, C. Photodynamic therapy in the management of potentially malignant and malignant oral disorders. *Head Neck Oncol.* **2012**, *4*, 16. [CrossRef]
54. Cerrati, E.W.; Nguyen, S.A.; Farrar, J.D.; Lentsch, E.J. The efficacy of photodynamic therapy in the treatment of oral squamous cell carcinoma: A meta-analysis. *Ent-Ear Nose Throat* **2015**, *94*, 72–79. [CrossRef] [PubMed]
55. Hinger, D.; Grafe, S.; Navarro, F.; Spingler, B.; Pandiarajan, D.; Walt, H.; Couffin, A.C.; Maake, C. Lipid nanoemulsions and liposomes improve photodynamic treatment efficacy and tolerance in CAL-33 tumor bearing nude mice. *J. Nanobiotechnol.* **2016**, *14*, 71. [CrossRef]
56. Piskorz, J.; Skupin, P.; Lijewski, S.; Korpusinski, M.; Sciepura, M.; Konopka, K.; Sobiak, S.; Goslinski, T.; Mielcarek, J. Synthesis, physical-chemical properties and in vitro photodynamic activity against oral cancer cells of novel porphyrazines possessing fluoroalkylthio and dietherthio substituents. *J. Fluor. Chem.* **2012**, *135*, 265–271. [CrossRef]
57. Piskorz, J.; Konopka, K.; Düzgüneş, N.; Gdaniec, Z.; Mielcarek, J.; Goslinski, T. Diazepinoporphyrazines containing peripheral styryl substituents and their promising nanomolar photodynamic activity against oral cancer cells in liposomal formulations. *Chemmedchem* **2014**, *9*, 1775–1782. [CrossRef]
58. Neves, S.; Faneca, H.; Bertin, S.; Konopka, K.; Düzgüneş, N.; Pierrefite-Carle, V.; Simoes, S.; de Lima, M.C.P. Transferrin lipoplex-mediated suicide gene therapy of oral squamous cell carcinoma in an immunocompetent murine model and mechanisms involved in the antitumoral response. *Cancer Gene Ther.* **2009**, *16*, 91–101. [CrossRef]
59. Liu, J.J.; Tian, L.L.; Zhang, R.; Dong, Z.L.; Wang, H.R.; Liu, Z. Collagenase-encapsulated pH-responsive nanoscale coordination polymers for tumor microenvironment modulation and enhanced photodynamic nanomedicine. *ACS Appl. Mater. Inter.* **2018**, *10*, 43493–43502. [CrossRef] [PubMed]
60. Kohli, A.G.; Kivimae, S.; Tiffany, M.R.; Szoka, F.C. Improving the distribution of Doxil (R) in the tumor matrix by depletion of tumor hyaluronan. *J. Control Release* **2014**, *191*, 105–114. [CrossRef]
61. Dolor, A.; Szoka, F.C. Digesting a path forward: The Uutility of collagenase tumor treatment for improved drug delivery. *Mol. Pharmaceut.* **2018**, *15*, 2069–2083. [CrossRef]
62. Pandey, M.; Choudhury, H.; Ying, J.N.S.; Ling, J.F.S.; Ting, J.; Ting, J.S.S.; Hwen, I.K.Z.; Suen, H.W.; Kamar, H.S.S.; Gorain, B.; et al. Mucoadhesive nanocarriers as a promising strategy to enhance intracellular delivery against oral cavity carcinoma. *Pharmaceutics* **2022**, *14*, 795. [CrossRef]
63. Alaei, S.; Omidian, H. Mucoadhesion and mechanical assessment of oral films. *Eur. J. Pharm. Sci.* **2021**, *159*, 105727. [CrossRef] [PubMed]
64. Piskorz, J.; Lijewski, S.; Gierszewski, M.; Gorniak, K.; Sobotta, L.; Wicher, B.; Tykarska, E.; Duzgunes, N.; Konopka, K.; Sikorski, D.; et al. Sulfanyl porphyrazines: Molecular barrel-like self-assembly in crystals, optical properties and in vitro photodynamic activity towards cancer cells. *Dyes Pigment.* **2017**, *136*, 898–908. [CrossRef]
65. Skupin-Mrugalska, P.; Koczorowski, T.; Szczolko, W.; Dlugaszewska, J.; Teubert, A.; Piotrowska-Kempisty, H.; Goslinski, T.; Sobotta, L. Cationic porphyrazines with morpholinoethyl substituents-Syntheses, optical properties, and photocytotoxicities. *Dyes Pigment.* **2022**, *197*, 109937. [CrossRef]
66. Mlynarczyk, D.T.; Lijewski, S.; Falkowski, M.; Piskorz, J.; Szczolko, W.; Sobotta, L.; Stolarska, M.; Popenda, L.; Jurga, S.; Konopka, K.; et al. Dendrimeric sulfanyl porphyrazines: Synthesis, physico-chemical characterization, and biological activity for potential applications in photodynamic therapy. *Chempluschem* **2016**, *81*, 460–470. [CrossRef] [PubMed]
67. Mlynarczyk, D.T.; Piskorz, J.; Popenda, L.; Stolarska, M.; Szczolko, W.; Konopka, K.; Jurga, S.; Sobotta, L.; Mielcarek, J.; Düzgüneş, N.; et al. S-seco-porphyrazine as a new member of the seco-porphyrazine family-Synthesis, characterization and photocytotoxicity against cancer cells. *Bioorg. Chem.* **2020**, *96*, 103634. [CrossRef]
68. Piskorz, J.; Mlynarczyk, D.T.; Szczolko, W.; Konopka, K.; Düzgüneş, N.; Mielcarek, J. Liposomal formulations of magnesium sulfanyl tribenzoporphyrazines for the photodynamic therapy of cancer. *J. Inorg. Biochem.* **2018**, *184*, 34–41. [CrossRef]
69. Young, M.; Yee, M.; Kim, H.Y.; Cheung, J.; Chino, T.; Düzgüneş, N.; Konopka, K. Phototoxicity of liposomal Zn-and Al-phthalocyanine against cervical and oral squamous cell carcinoma cells in vitro. *Med. Sci. Monit. Basic* **2016**, *22*, 156–164. [CrossRef]
70. Cheung, J.; Furukawa, D.; Pandez, R.; Yıldırım, M.; Frazier, A.; Piskorz, J.; Düzgüneş, N.; Konopka, K. Photocytotoxicity of liposomal zinc phthalocyanine in oral squamous cell carcinoma and pharyngeal carcinoma cells. *Ther. Deliv.* **2020**, *11*, 547–556. [CrossRef] [PubMed]
71. Skupin-Mrugalska, P.; Szczolko, W.; Gierlich, P.; Konopka, K.; Goslinski, T.; Mielcarek, J.; Düzgüneş, N. Physicochemical properties of liposome-incorporated 2-(morpholin-4-yl)ethoxy phthalocyanines and their photodynamic activity against oral cancer cells. *J. Photoch. Photobio. A* **2018**, *353*, 445–457. [CrossRef]

72. Dlugaszewska, J.; Szczolko, W.; Koczorowski, T.; Skupin-Mrugalska, P.; Teubert, A.; Konopka, K.; Kucinska, M.; Murias, M.; Düzgüneş, N.; Mielcarek, J.; et al. Antimicrobial and anticancer photodynamic activity of a phthalocyanine photosensitizer with N-methyl morpholiniumethoxy substituents in non-peripheral positions. *J. Inorg. Biochem.* **2017**, *172*, 67–79. [CrossRef] [PubMed]
73. Janas, K.; Boniewska-Bernacka, E.; Dyrda, G.; Slota, R. Porphyrin and phthalocyanine photosensitizers designed for targeted photodynamic therapy of colorectal cancer. *Bioorgan. Med. Chem.* **2021**, *30*, 115926. [CrossRef] [PubMed]
74. Santos, K.L.M.; Barros, R.M.; Lima, D.P.S.; Nunes, A.M.A.; Sato, M.R.; Faccio, R.; Damasceno, B.P.G.D.; Oshiro, J.A. Prospective application of phthalocyanines in the photodynamic therapy against microorganisms and tumor cells: A mini-review. *Photodiagn. Photodyn.* **2020**, *32*, 102032. [CrossRef] [PubMed]
75. Thomas, A.P.; Babu, P.S.S.; Nair, S.A.; Ramakrishnan, S.; Ramaiah, D.; Chandrashekar, T.K.; Srinivasan, A.; Pillai, M.R. meso-Tetrakis(p-sulfonatophenyl)N-confused porphyrin tetrasodium salt: A potential sensitizer for photodynamic therapy. *J. Med. Chem.* **2012**, *55*, 5110–5120. [CrossRef] [PubMed]
76. Chin, Y.; Lim, S.H.; Zorlu, Y.; Ahsen, V.; Kiew, L.V.; Chung, L.Y.; Dumoulin, F.; Lee, H.B. Improved photodynamic efficacy of Zn(II) phthalocyanines via glycerol substitution. *PLoS ONE* **2014**, *9*, e97894. [CrossRef]
77. Moon, S.; Bae, J.Y.; Son, H.K.; Lee, D.Y.; Park, G.; You, H.; Ko, H.; Kim, Y.C.; Kim, J. RUNX3 confers sensitivity to pheophorbide a-photodynamic therapy in human oral squamous cell carcinoma cell lines. *Laser Med. Sci.* **2015**, *30*, 499–507. [CrossRef]
78. Chu, P.L.; Shihabuddeen, W.A.; Low, K.P.; Poon, D.J.J.; Ramaswamy, B.; Lang, Z.G.; Nei, W.L.; Chua, K.L.M.; Thong, P.S.P.; Soo, K.C.; et al. Vandetanib sensitizes head and neck squamous cell carcinoma to photodynamic therapy through modulation of EGFR-dependent DNA repair and the tumour microenvironment. *Photodiagn. Photodyn.* **2019**, *27*, 367–374. [CrossRef]
79. Bonnet, D.; Dick, J.E. Human acute myeloid leukemia is organized as a hierarchy that originates from a primitive hematopoietic cell. *Nat. Med.* **1997**, *3*, 730–737. [CrossRef]
80. Al-Hajj, M.; Wicha, M.S.; Benito-Hernandez, A.; Morrison, S.J.; Clarke, M.F. Prospective identification of tumorigenic breast cancer cells. *Proc. Natl. Acad. Sci. USA* **2003**, *100*, 3983–3988. [CrossRef]
81. Mackenzie, I.C. Growth of malignant oral epithelial stem cells after seeding into organotypical cultures of normal mucosa. *J. Oral Pathol. Med.* **2004**, *33*, 71–78. [CrossRef]
82. Mannelli, G.; Gallo, O. Cancer stem cells hypothesis and stem cells in head and neck cancers. *Cancer Treat. Rev.* **2012**, *38*, 515–539. [CrossRef]
83. Rodini, C.O.; Lopes, N.M.; Lara, V.S.; Mackenzie, I.C. Oral cancer stem cells-properties and consequences. *J. Appl. Oral Sci.* **2017**, *25*, 708–715. [CrossRef] [PubMed]
84. Elkashty, O.A.; Abu Elghanam, G.; Su, X.Y.; Liu, Y.N.; Chauvin, P.J.; Tran, S.D. Cancer stem cells enrichment with surface markers CD271 and CD44 in human head and neck squamous cell carcinomas. *Carcinogenesis* **2020**, *41*, 458–466. [CrossRef] [PubMed]
85. Güleryüz, B.; Ünal, U.; Gülsoy, M. Near infrared light activated upconversion nanoparticles (UCNP) based photodynamic therapy of prostate cancers: An in vitro study. *Photodiagn. Photodyn. Ther.* **2021**, *36*, 102616. [CrossRef]
86. Chatterjee, D.K.; Yong, Z. Upconverting nanoparticles as nanotransducers for photodynamic therapy in cancer cells. *Nanomedicine* **2008**, *3*, 73–82. [CrossRef] [PubMed]
87. Sawamura, T.; Tanaka, T.; Ishige, H.; Iizuka, M.; Murayama, Y.; Otsuji, E.; Ohkubo, A.; Ogura, S.I.; Yuasa, H. The effect of coatings on the affinity of lanthanide nanoparticles to MKN45 and HeLa cancer cells and improvement in photodynamic therapy Eeficiency. *Int. J. Mol. Sci.* **2015**, *16*, 22415–22424. [CrossRef]
88. Wang, B.Y.; Liao, M.L.; Hong, G.C.; Chang, W.W.; Chu, C.C. Near-infrared-triggered photodynamic therapy toward breast cancer cells using dendrimer-functionalized upconversion nanoparticles. *Nanomaterials* **2017**, *7*, 269. [CrossRef] [PubMed]
89. Wan, Y.L.; Fu, L.H.; Li, C.Y.; Lin, J.; Huang, P. Conquering the hypoxia limitation for photodynamic therapy. *Adv. Mater.* **2021**, *33*, 202103978. [CrossRef]

Disclaimer/Publisher's Note: The statements, opinions and data contained in all publications are solely those of the individual author(s) and contributor(s) and not of MDPI and/or the editor(s). MDPI and/or the editor(s) disclaim responsibility for any injury to people or property resulting from any ideas, methods, instructions or products referred to in the content.

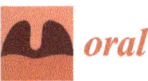

Opinion

Skeletal Anchorage in Treating Skeletal Class II Malocclusion in Growing Patients Using the Herbst Appliance

Antonio Manni [1], Stefano Pera [2,*], Giorgio Gastaldi [2], Andrea Boggio [2] and Mauro Cozzani [3]

1. Private Practice, 73055 Racale, LE, Italy; dottantoniomanni@gmail.com
2. Dental School, Vita-Salute San Raffaele University, 20132 Milan, MI, Italy; gastaldi.giorgio@hsr.it (G.G.); andreaboggio90@gmail.com (A.B.)
3. Istituto Giuseppe Cozzani, 19125 La Spezia, SP, Italy; maurocozzani@gmail.com
* Correspondence: pe.ste.97@live.it

Abstract: Skeletal Class II is a common malocclusion affecting the Caucasian population and characterized, in most cases, by a convex profile and mandibular retrusion. Therefore, the treatment plan often requires the use of functional appliances to promote mandibular advancement. In particular, the Herbst appliance is recommended because of its efficiency and minimal need for compliance. However, in addition to skeletal favorable effects, undesired dental compensations could prematurely reduce the overjet needed for a proper orthopedic outcome. The combination of this appliance with skeletal anchorage and elastic ligatures in the lower or both, in the upper and the lower arch, enables effective control of unfavorable tooth movements, improving the therapeutic potential of such a treatment. These improvements have significantly shifted the main focus on facial aesthetics rather than dental occlusion, with the creation of innovative treatment protocols and a new diagnostic approach to Class II malocclusion.

Keywords: Herbst; Class II; TADS; facial esthetics

1. Introduction

Class II malocclusion is a common occlusal disorder in the Caucasian population, characterized by a convex facial profile and caused by a combination of skeletal and dental components, each of which contributes to its characteristics and severity. Only a small percentage of cases exhibit maxillary skeletal protrusion. On the average, the maxilla is in a neutral position or even retruded, while the mandible is mostly retruded [1].

So, the correction of dento-skeletal Class II malocclusion requires a comprehensive evaluation that includes both qualitative and quantitative analysis of the deviated elements. In addition to general diagnostic records such as photograph and radiograph, Fränkel's maneuver [2] is a crucial tool in this process, as it provides a clinical assessment of the subject and helps to identify the deviated elements.

The Fränkel maneuver involves protracting the mandible with half-closed lips until a proper canine Class I is achieved. The patient is then asked to close their lips, and the change in profile is evaluated to determine the most appropriate treatment strategy which may involve advancing the mandible, retracting the upper jaw, or a combination of both. However, this maneuver is based on occlusion, with the main focus on achieving a proper dental relation and only later evaluating the patient's esthetics. This might be so because traditional therapies have limitations as they primarily affect the dentoalveolar component (70%) and only partially the skeletal component (30%) [3,4]. These limitations are due to anchorage loss with sagittal and vertical tooth movements, which are common with most of orthodontic appliances (proclination of lower incisors, lingual inclination of upper incisors, and clockwise rotation of the occlusal plane).

Indeed, a conventional functional treatment include a Pogonion advancement of at best 2 mm, a maxillary retraction of 1 mm, and a clockwise rotation of the mandibular

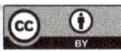

plane (1° on average) [5]. However, this might result in some cases in an aesthetically unacceptable correction, especially when a greater mandibular advancement is required, and maxillary retraction is undesirable.

Another critical factor in treating Class II malocclusions in growing patients is the overjet. In an ideal occlusion, the overjet is defined as the distance between the buccal surface of the lower central incisor and the palatal surface of the upper one. However, in the presence of a Class II malocclusion, the overjet might be considered as the minimum distance between the buccal surface of the lower six front teeth and the palatal surface of the upper ones, which is usable for mandibular advancement.

In fact, the extent of mandibular advancement will depend mainly on the initial overjet and the ability to maintain or increase it during the treatment [6]. Therapies involving a large initial overjet or having the potential to create one (such as proclination of the incisors for correction of Class II Division II) are likely to achieve a significant mandibular advancement, with a high probability of success [7].

2. Compliance

The success of Class II correction therapy also depends on patient cooperation. While numerous therapies have been proposed, including fixed and removable functional appliances and Class II elastics, patient compliance is known to be a challenge (in many cases, compliance is estimated to be between 27 and 37% for treatments that rely on the patient) [8–11]. Considering this, fixed functional appliances, such as the Herbst appliance, are particularly valuable in achieving a successful outcome.

3. Notes on Skeletal and Dentolaveolar Effects

Despite its original design [12] being limited to severe Class II malocclusions and uncooperative patients, the clinical management of Herbst appliance has been modified in recent years and now boasts a higher success rate.

The traditional Herbst appliance, like other functional devices including Class II elastics, has both dentoalveolar and skeletal effects related to direction of the applied forces [13]. The distalization of the upper arch and a slowdown in the forward growth of the maxilla (by approximately -0.4 to 1 mm due to the extraoral traction effect) [14,15] are combined with mesialization of the lower arch and mandibular advancement, resulting in a statistically significant but clinically insignificant Pog advancement of 1.45 to 1.91 mm [16]. Alveolodental movements, caused by a reciprocal loss of anchorage, are more prevalent (70–80%) compared to skeletal movements (20–30%), with variations depending on the treatment period (pre-peak, peak, post-peak) and the extent of the original malocclusion.

So, the skeletal effects of the Herbst appliance are limited by the alveolodental movements in both the vertical and sagittal planes [16–18]. In the upper arch, the molars intrude and distalize, while the incisors extrude and lingualize (by approximately 1.5 to 3.5 mm on average) [14,15]; in the lower arch, the molars extrude and mesialize and the incisors intrude and buccally flare (with an average proclination of 7.5 to 10.5°) [5,7]. This results in a rapid overjet reduction and a clockwise rotation of the occlusal plane and of the mandible, losing some of the mandibular advancement.

This effect can be controlled with the use of a full-coverage resin splint, making Herbst therapy possible even for patients with increased vertical dimension and improving the anchorage, although the results are partial.

4. The Skeletal Anchorage

If the movement of teeth interfere with the sagittal advancement of the mandible, reducing these movements with skeletal anchorage could result in a better Class II aesthetic correction.

Anchorage in the lower arch involves the use of a resin splint, buccal miniscrews, and elastic ligatures (Figures 1 and 2). The miniscrews are placed bilaterally between the first molar and second lower premolar, with the head positioned in the attached gingiva or on the mucogingival line. Two bondable buttons are placed on the buccal surface of the canines and connected to the miniscrews through elastic ligatures of 150–200 g. This configuration, combined with the splint, prevents molar mesialization and proclination of the incisors and enables effective control of the entire arch. The elastic ligatures should be parallel to the occlusal plane and replaced every 4 weeks. In addition, splinting the lower six frontal elements can prevent rotation, distalization, and intrusion of the canines caused by elastic traction.

This technique results in a greater skeletal effect, an average reduction in the gonial angle by 1.3–1.5°, a counterclockwise rotation of the mandible, and greater advancement of the Pog of 3.8–4.0 mm [19,20].

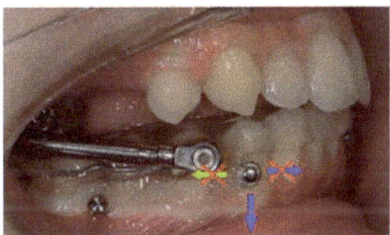

Figure 1. Right lateral view of anchorage in the lower arch.

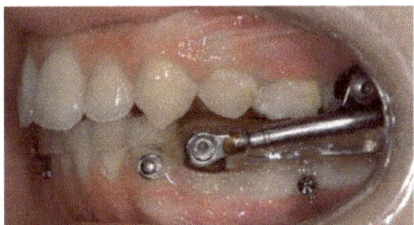

Figure 2. Left lateral view of anchorage in the lower arch.

Moreover, when distalization of the upper arch with opening of Nasolabial angle is undesired, a similar anchorage reinforcement is required also in the upper arch (Figures 3 and 4). The arch is stabilized by the fixed appliances, with the transverse dimension blocked by the palatal arch of the Herbst appliance. The miniscrews are placed bilaterally between the first premolar and canine or, in some cases, between the second and first premolar. Elastic ligatures are stretched from the miniscrews to first molar bands, in a horizontal direction. This configuration reduces distalization of the molars and lingualization of the upper incisors, preserving the overjet, limiting the opening of nasolabial angle, and improving the aesthetic outcome also in biretruded Class II patients.

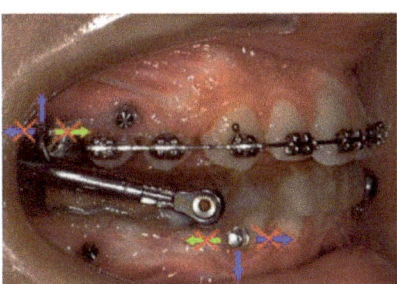

Figure 3. Right lateral view of anchorage in the upper arch.

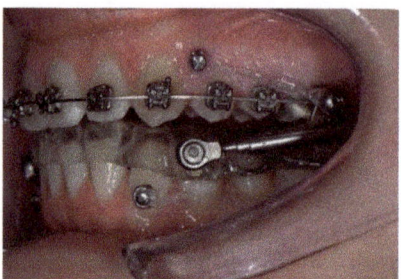

Figure 4. Left lateral view of anchorage in the upper arch.

To date, a pilot study showed an average Pog advancement of 5.7 mm with the use of Herbst MTH, 4 buccal miniscrews, and elastic ligatures [20].

Moreover, anchorage in the upper arch can be similarly managed using palatal miniscrews instead of buccal ones, increasing the potential of the technique.

5. A New Diagnostic Approach

Skeletal anchorage has increased the percentage of skeletal correction from 30 to 70%, with the ability to selectively modify individual components of the Class II malocclusion [19,20]. Traditional techniques facilitate the retraction of the maxilla or simultaneous retraction of the maxilla and advancement of the mandible, but not separately and not in a clinically significant manner. With the addition of skeletal anchorage, it is now possible to selectively (a) retract the maxilla; (b) advance the maxilla; (c) retract the maxilla and advance the mandible in a clinically significant manner; and (d) advance the mandible in a clinically significant manner.

This has led to a new diagnostic approach, considering more facial aesthetics rather than occlusal relation. As a result, Fränkel's maneuver has been modified with a new maneuver known as Manni's Aesthetic maneuver, which places most importance on aesthetics: basically, the patient is asked to bring the mandible forward until an aesthetically optimal position is achieved with closed lips (not open as in traditional Fränkel's maneuver). Only after he is asked to open the lips to evaluate the occlusal relation. So, the decision of the optimal skeletal position is based on aesthetic0073 rather than occlusion, with much emphasis placed on the nasolabial angle, lips, maxillary, and mandibular sagittal position, evaluated through clinical and photographic analysis.

6. Conclusions

- A proper Skeletal Class II treatment requires specific focus on patient aesthetics.
- Skeletal anchorage facilitates a reduction in dental compensations and increased skeletal effects of orthopedic therapy [21,22].
- The combination of the Herbst MTH appliance with elastic ligatures and skeletal anchorage in the lower, or both lower and upper arch, represent an effective and efficient therapy in the management of Class II malocclusion, with the possibility of modulating the effects on the maxilla and mandible.
- The presence of a mandibular splint provides increased control of verticality and limits post-rotation of the occlusal and mandibular plane, with significant effects on Pogonion projection [23].
- Achieving and maintaining a functional overjet to the mandibular advancement is the key to a successful treatment.

However, these conclusions should be interpreted with caution, as currently available research is not enough appropriate to determine the long-term effects of such a treatment, and further well-designed randomized clinical trials are needed to confirm these results.

Author Contributions: Conceptualization, A.M. and A.B.; methodology, A.M. and A.B.; software, S.P.; validation, A.M., M.C. and G.G.; formal analysis, A.B. and S.P.; investigation, A.M.; resources, A.M.; writing—original draft preparation, S.P.; writing—review and editing, A.B.; visualization, S.P.; supervision, M.C. and G.G.; project administration, G.G. and M.C. All authors have read and agreed to the published version of the manuscript.

Funding: This research received no external funding.

Institutional Review Board Statement: Ethical review and approval were waived for this study since it turns out to be an opinion.

Data Availability Statement: Not applicable.

Conflicts of Interest: The authors declare no conflict of interest.

References

1. McNamara, J.A., Jr. Components of Class II malocclusion in children 8–10 years of age. *Angle Orthod.* **1981**, *51*, 177–202. [CrossRef] [PubMed]
2. Fränkel, R.; Fränkel, C. *Orofacial Orthopedics with the Function Regulator*; Karger Publishers: Basel, Switzerland, 1989.
3. Bock, N.C.; Gnandt, E.; Ruf, S. Occlusal stability after Herbst treatment of patients with retrognathic and prognathic facial types: A pilot study. *J. Orofac. Orthop.* **2016**, *77*, 160–167. [CrossRef] [PubMed]
4. VanLaecken, R.; Martin, C.A.; Dischinger, T.; Razmus, T.; Ngan, P. Treatment effects of the edgewise Herbst appliance: A cephalometric and tomographic investigation. *Am. J. Orthod. Dentofac. Orthop.* **2006**, *130*, 582–593. [CrossRef] [PubMed]
5. Valant, J.R.; Sinclair, P.M. Treatment effects of the Herbst appliance. *Am. J. Orthod. Dentofac. Orthop.* **1989**, *95*, 138–147. [CrossRef] [PubMed]
6. Pancherz, H. The Herbst appliance—Its biologic effects and clinical use. *Am. J. Orthod.* **1985**, *87*, 1–20. [CrossRef] [PubMed]
7. Casutt, C.; Pancherz, H.; Gawora, M.; Ruf, S. Success rate and efficiency of activator treatment. *Eur. J. Orthod.* **2007**, *29*, 614–621. [CrossRef] [PubMed]
8. Čirgić, E.; Kjellberg, H.; Hansen, K. Treatment of large overjet in Angle Class II: Division 1 malocclusion with Andresen activators versus prefabricated functional appliances—A multicenter, randomized, controlled trial. *Eur. J. Orthod.* **2016**, *38*, 516–524. [CrossRef]
9. Arreghini, A.; Trigila, S.; Lombardo, L.; Siciliani, G. Objective assessment of compliance with intra- and extraoral removable appliances. *Angle Orthod.* **2017**, *87*, 88–95. [CrossRef]
10. Veeroo, H.J.; Cunningham, S.J.; Newton, J.T.; Travess, H.C. Motivation and compliance with intraoral elastics. *Am. J. Orthod. Dentofac. Orthop.* **2014**, *146*, 33–39. [CrossRef]
11. Schiöth, T.; Von Bremen, J.; Pancherz, H.; Ruf, S. Complications during Herbst Appliance Treatment with Reduced Mandibular Cast Splints: A prospective, clinical multicenter study. *J. Orofac. Orthop.* **2007**, *68*, 321–327. [CrossRef]
12. Pancherz, H. The mechanism of Class II correction in Herbst appliance treatment: A cephalometric investigation. *Am. J. Orthod.* **1982**, *82*, 104–113. [CrossRef] [PubMed]
13. LeCornu, M.; Cevidanes, L.H.; Zhu, H.; Wu, C.-D.; Larson, B.; Nguyen, T. Three-dimensional treatment outcomes in Class II patients treated with the Herbst appliance: A pilot study. *Am. J. Orthod. Dentofac. Orthop.* **2013**, *144*, 818–830. [CrossRef] [PubMed]
14. Pancherz, H.; Fackel, U. The skeletofacial growth pattern pre-and post-dentofacial orthopaedics. A long-term study of Class II malocclusions treated with the Herbst appliance. *Eur. J. Orthod.* **1990**, *12*, 209–218. [CrossRef] [PubMed]
15. Yang, X.; Zhu, Y.; Long, H.; Zhou, Y.; Jian, F.; Ye, N.; Gao, M.; Lai, W. The effectiveness of the Herbst appliance for patients with Class II malocclusion: A meta-analysis. *Eur. J. Orthod.* **2016**, *38*, 324–333. [CrossRef] [PubMed]
16. Sangalli, K.L.; Dutra-Horstmann, K.L.; Correr, G.M.; Topolski, F.; Flores-Mir, C.; Lagravère, M.O.; Moro, A. Three-dimensional skeletal and dentoalveolar sagittal and vertical changes associated with cantilever Herbst appliance in prepubertal patients with Class II malocclusion. *Am. J. Orthod. Dentofac. Orthop.* **2022**, *161*, 638–651.e1. [CrossRef] [PubMed]
17. Hägg, U.; Pancherz, H. Dentofacial orthopaedics in relation to chronological age, growth period and skeletal development. An analysis of 72 male patients with Class II division 1 malocclusion treated with the Herbst appliance. *Eur. J. Orthod.* **1988**, *10*, 169–176. [CrossRef]
18. Manni, A.; Mutinelli, S.; Cerruto, C.; Cozzani, M. Influence of incisor position control on the mandibular response in growing patients with skeletal Class II malocclusion. *Am. J. Orthod. Dentofac. Orthop.* **2021**, *159*, 594–603. [CrossRef]
19. Manni, A.; Mutinelli, S.; Pasini, M.; Mazzotta, L.; Cozzani, M. Herbst appliance anchored to miniscrews with 2 types of ligation: Effectiveness in skeletal Class II treatment. *Am. J. Orthod. Dentofac. Orthop.* **2016**, *149*, 871–880. [CrossRef]
20. Manni, A.; Migliorati, M.; Calzolari, C.; Silvestrini-Biavati, A. Herbst appliance anchored to miniscrews in the upper and lower arches vs standard Herbst: A pilot study. *Am. J. Orthod. Dentofac. Orthop.* **2019**, *156*, 617–625. [CrossRef]
21. Al-Dboush, R.; Soltan, R.; Rao, J.; El-Bialy, T. Skeletal and dental effects of Herbst appliance anchored with temporary anchorage devices: A systematic review with meta-analysis. *Orthod. Craniofacial Res.* **2021**, *25*, 31–48. [CrossRef]

22. Huang, Y.; Sun, W.; Xiong, X.; Zhang, Z.; Liu, J.; Wang, J. Effects of fixed functional appliances with temporary anchorage devices on Class II malocclusion: A systematic review and meta-analysis. *J. World Fed. Orthod.* **2021**, *10*, 59–69. [CrossRef] [PubMed]
23. Manni, A.; Pasini, M.; Mazzotta, L.; Mutinelli, S.; Nuzzo, C.; Grassi, F.R.; Cozzani, M. Comparison between an Acrylic Splint Herbst and an Acrylic Splint Miniscrew-Herbst for Mandibular Incisors Proclination Control. *Int. J. Dent.* **2014**, *2014*, 173187. [CrossRef] [PubMed]

Disclaimer/Publisher's Note: The statements, opinions and data contained in all publications are solely those of the individual author(s) and contributor(s) and not of MDPI and/or the editor(s). MDPI and/or the editor(s) disclaim responsibility for any injury to people or property resulting from any ideas, methods, instructions or products referred to in the content.

MDPI AG
Grosspeteranlage 5
4052 Basel
Switzerland
Tel.: +41 61 683 77 34

Oral Editorial Office
E-mail: oral@mdpi.com
www.mdpi.com/journal/oral

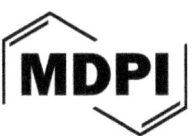

Disclaimer/Publisher's Note: The statements, opinions and data contained in all publications are solely those of the individual author(s) and contributor(s) and not of MDPI and/or the editor(s). MDPI and/or the editor(s) disclaim responsibility for any injury to people or property resulting from any ideas, methods, instructions or products referred to in the content.

www.ingramcontent.com/pod-product-compliance
Lightning Source LLC
LaVergne TN
LVHW070045120526
838202LV00101B/434